World Health Organization

REGIONAL OFFICE FOR Europe

Health 2020
A European policy framework and strategy for the 21st century

Abstract

The 53 countries of the European Region approved a new value- and evidence-based health policy framework for the Region, Health 2020, at the session of the WHO Regional Committee for Europe in September 2012. Health 2020 focuses on improving health for all and reducing health inequalities, through improved leadership and governance for health. It focuses on today's major health problems. It identifies four priority areas for policy action and is innovative in terms of responses across all levels and sectors of government and society, emphasizing developing assets and resilience within communities, empowerment and creating supportive environments. It details the strengthened roles of public health services and the health system. Health 2020 was approved in two forms: a European policy framework supporting action across government and society for health and well-being for politicians and those developing policy and the longer Health 2020 policy framework and strategy, which provides more operational detail. Implementing Health 2020 in countries is now the fundamental top-priority challenge for the Region.

Keywords

HEALTH POLICY
HEALTH SYSTEMS PLANS
DELIVERY OF HEALTH CARE
REGIONAL HEALTH PLANNING
INTERNATIONAL COOPERATION
PUBLIC HEALTH
EUROPE

ISBN 978 92 890 0279 0

Address requests about publications of the WHO Regional Office for Europe to:
Publications
WHO Regional Office for Europe
UN City
Marmorvej 51
DK-2100 Copenhagen Ø, Denmark
Alternatively, complete an online request form for documentation, health information, or for permission to quote or translate, on the Regional Office web site (http://www.euro.who.int/pubrequest).

Book design and cover design: Christophe Lanoux, Paris, France

Contents

Introduction 1

Health 2020: a European policy framework supporting action across government and society for health and well-being 5

Health 2020: policy framework and strategy 25

Introduction

Health 2020 is a value- and evidence-based health policy framework for health and well-being among the people of the WHO European Region. The hope is that Health 2020 will provide understanding and inspiration to everyone across the European Region who wishes to seize new opportunities to improve the health and well-being of present and future generations, by showing both the challenges, opportunities and ways forward. Health 2020 is for everyone: not just politicians and experts but also civil society, communities, families and individuals.

Why is Health 2020 important? Health 2020 presents the social and economic imperative for action, showing clearly that health and well-being are important and essential for economic and social development. It focuses on health as a human right; whole-of-government and whole-of-society approaches to equitable improvement in health; strong and invigorated governance and leadership for health; collaborative models of working and shared priorities with other sectors; the importance of community and individual reliance and empowerment; and the role of partnerships.

The WHO Regional Committee for Europe approved Health 2020 in 2012 in two documentary forms, included here in a single publication. The European policy framework for supporting government and society for health and well-being provides politicians and policy practitioners with the main values and principles needed to put Health 2020 into practice. It focuses on today's major health challenges as well as the opportunities for equitable improvement in health and provides strong political, social and economic arguments for health action, built around the policy framework's key strategic policy objectives and priorities.

The longer Health 2020 policy framework and strategy provides in much greater detail the contextual analysis and the main strategies and interventions that work as well as the necessary evidence and details of the capacity required for implementing the policies and practices designed to improve health and well-being. The emphasis is on innovative and evidence-informed policy and practice, presented to assist those who develop and implement operational policy. The Health 2020 policy framework and strategy is seen as a living guide, providing links to later changes in evidence, practice and outcomes.

Taken together, these publications provide a flexible framework for policy and practice across the Member States of the European Region, building on a long history of global and regional policy thinking. Health 2020 is fully aligned with the WHO reform process and will be actively promoted by the WHO Regional Office for Europe among its Member States, who should receive integrated in-country support in the context of their individual needs and priorities. Here WHO must work in partnership, and everyone involved in developing Health 2020 must be willing to advocate for it and be committed to make it work.

Health 2020: a European policy framework supporting action across government and society for health and well-being

Contents

Foreword ... 8

Foreword ... 9

Health is a major societal resource and asset ... 11

A strong value base: reaching the highest attainable standard of health ... 12

A strong social and economic case for improving health ... 12

Strategic objectives of Health 2020: stronger equity and better governance for health ... 13

Improving health for all and reducing health inequalities ... 13

Improving leadership and participatory governance for health ... 14

Working together on common policy priorities for health ... 15

Priority area 1. Investing in health through a life-course approach and empowering people ... 16

Priority area 2. Tackling Europe's major health challenges: noncommunicable and communicable diseases ... 17

Priority area 3. Strengthening people-centred health systems, public health capacity and emergency preparedness, surveillance and response ... 18

Priority area 4. Creating resilient communities and supportive environments ... 20

Working together: adding value through partnerships ... 20

Health 2020 – a common purpose and a shared responsibility ... 22

Foreword

Health 2020: a European policy framework supporting action across government and society for health and well-being sets out a far-sighted and ambitious agenda for health. Agreement on this framework by all 53 Member States of the WHO European Region comes at a crucial time. As we approach 2015 and the deadline for achieving the Millennium Development Goals, this policy will help to position health in the next generation of global goals.

The framework crystallizes what we have learned about the role of health in recent years. Maximizing health through all stages of life is a fundamental right for all and not a privilege for a few. Good health is an asset and a source of economic and social stability. It is key to reducing poverty and both contributes to and benefits from sustainable development. Most important, good health can no longer be seen an outcome of one sector alone: sustainable and equitable improvements in health are the product of effective policy across all parts of government and collaborative efforts across all parts of society.

Readers will find that these insights lie at the heart of the strategy. The challenges to be addressed in the Region are considerable. Health inequities within and between countries reflect economic and social divisions across society. As economic pressures bite and health care costs rise, the risk of exclusion increases, too often leaving behind those with the greatest health needs. At the same time, we know that public expectations for the newest and the best in health technology in combination with the changing disease profile of ageing populations place huge pressure on budgets. New approaches and perspectives are needed if universal health coverage is to be a reality for the countries of the Region. Shifting the mindset of policy-makers, health providers and members of the public from one that sees health in terms of combating illness to one mainly focusing on promoting health and well-being is the key to the future. Success requires political support, technical and administrative innovation and changes in how financial resources and other assets are deployed.

The framework for Europe is closely aligned to WHO's Twelfth General Programme of Work and is a practical expression of a programme of reform in WHO that seeks to enable the Organization to respond to Member State needs more effectively in a rapidly changing world. In the European Region, as in other regions, the outcomes envisaged in this policy framework require that international organizations be able to work not just with selected sectoral ministries but across all relevant parts of government; with colleagues in other international organizations that influence health; as well as with industry, academe and civil society. The policy framework for Europe signals the way forward for new approaches to health and well-being worldwide.

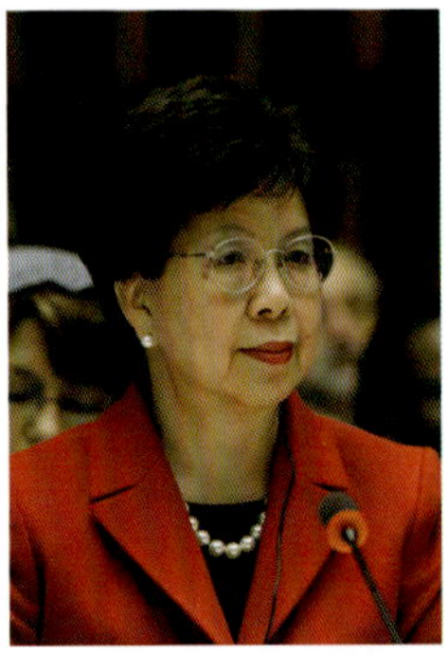

Margaret Chan
WHO Director-General

Foreword

It gives me great pleasure to welcome you to Health 2020, the European health policy framework for all. Whether you are a president, prime minister, mayor, policy-maker, public health worker or community activist, Health 2020 contains information that can help you make healthier, safer and economically wiser decisions and choices.

Our 21st century health landscape is shaped by growing global, regional, national and local interdependence and an increasingly complex array of interlinking factors that influence health and well-being. We are all challenged, for example, with the task of making sense of and integrating the many different actors and sectoral services (such as housing, water, energy, food and health care) needed to keep ourselves, our families and our populations healthy and happy. We all know that poor health wastes potential, causes despair and suffering and drains resources. Addressing these challenges at any level – personal, institutional, community, municipal or national – requires thoughtful, strategic and coordinated action. All 53 Member States in the WHO European Region have developed and adopted Health 2020 as a guiding framework to support such action.

Health 2020 elaborates a vision of public health as a dynamic network of stakeholders at all levels of society and aims to support action with unity of purpose across the Region. All recommendations in Health 2020 are evidence-informed. Its development has actively involved many experts. Our aim throughout has been to make Health 2020 a unique compilation of the best public health policy evidence available.

Building on an extensive review of published evidence, experiential data and an unprecedented Region-wide participatory stakeholder consultation, the Health 2020 development process has catalysed a broad rethinking of current public health mechanisms, processes, relationships and institutional arrangements. As a consequence of this process, Health 2020 serves as a unique regional resource to help us all learn from experiences acquired in practice, reset priorities and identify better ways to coordinate action amongst stakeholders in all sectors to improve individual and population health and well-being.

Health 2020 acknowledges and celebrates the wide diversity of health systems and approaches across the European Region. It aims not to make national and local health systems uniform but to make them uniformly better. In adopting Health 2020, all countries agreed on two common objectives: the need to improve health for all and reduce the health divide and the need to strengthen leadership and participatory governance for health.

In outlining ways to address these objectives, Health 2020 proposes new forms of governance for health, in which health and well-being are seen as the responsibility of the whole of society and of the whole of government, and encourages active public participation in policy-making.

It addresses the socioeconomic rationale for improving health and makes a strong, evidence-informed case for investment and action through integrated approaches to health promotion, disease prevention and well-being. Actions on social determinants are described that address the development of approaches that build health into all policies with the aim of improving the health of everyone and thereby reduce the absolute effect of social determinants on all people as well as targeted interventions that focus on those most affected.

Health 2020 identifies new systems of collaborative leadership to encourage innovative approaches to social mobilization for equitable, sustainable and accountable health development.

Health 2020 details a variety of innovative and effective ways to address today's complex public health challenges. It outlines a variety of strategies and interventions to address major health challenges across the lifespan related to both noncommunicable and infectious diseases. It shows ways to link clinical interventions with action on equity and social determinants of health and necessary key health system inputs such as human resources and medicines in higher quality, strengthening health funding arrangements and enhancing governance for health.

By articulating a common set of values, evidence and experience, Health 2020 provides a platform for partnership and cooperation. It calls for cross-society engagement as a central part of health policy planning, development, implementation and monitoring at all levels. It makes the case for empowering people, citizens, consumers and patients as a critical factor in improving health outcomes. It argues strongly for the engagement of health professionals.

What will WHO do to help? The Regional Office will support countries in adapting Health 2020 by analysing public health situations; identifying assets; encouraging political commitment from presidents and prime ministers; making policy recommendations and monitoring progress; encouraging leadership and good governance for health; suggesting mechanisms for whole-of-society and whole-of-government approaches; and supporting capacity development.

Two key Health 2020 support documents have been developed. The European policy framework for supporting government and society for health and well-being provides politicians, policy- and decision-makers and practitioners with the main values and action principles needed for putting a Health 2020 approach into practice in their settings. The longer Health 2020 policy framework and strategy provides more detail in terms of evidence and is meant for those who practice policy development and implementation at operational levels.

I believe Health 2020 can add significant value to all of our individual and collective work to enhance health and well-being, serve as unique resource to enhance the future and prosperity of individual countries and the Region as a whole and benefit all its peoples. Actively informing and aligning our daily practice with Health 2020 values and approaches will enable us to build a healthier Europe for ourselves and our children.

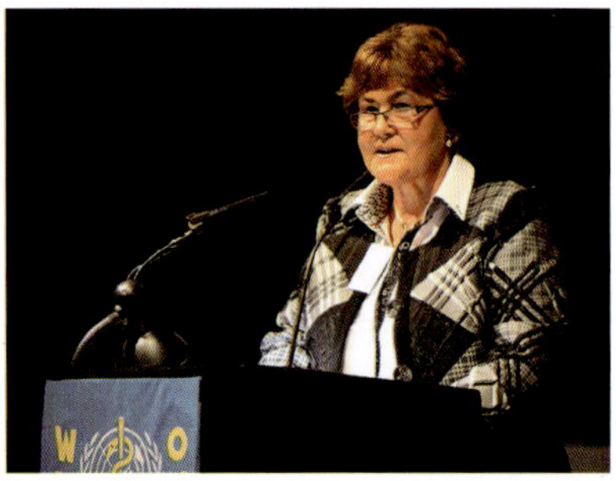

Zsuzsanna Jakab
WHO Regional Director for Europe

"The enjoyment of the highest attainable standard of health is one of the fundamental rights of every human being."

WHO Constitution

Dear Prime Minister, Minister, Mayor or Member of Parliament,

Good health underpins social and economic development and strengthens policies across all sectors. However, the economic and fiscal crisis facing many countries presents serious challenges and potentially risks undermining the positive progress that has been made. Nevertheless, it also presents an important opportunity to refocus and renew our efforts to improve the health of all people.

All sectors and levels of government contribute to health creation. **Your leadership for health and well-being can make a tremendous difference** for the people of your country, state, region or city and for the European Region as a whole.

Your support for Health 2020 is truly essential.

"We want to see better health and well-being for all, as an equal human right. Money does not buy better health. Good policies that promote equity have a better chance. We must tackle the root causes (of ill health and inequities) through a social determinants approach that engages the whole of government and the whole of society."

Margaret Chan,
WHO Director-General

The 53 Member States in the WHO European Region have agreed on a new common policy framework – **Health 2020. Their shared goals are to "significantly improve the health and well-being of populations, reduce health inequalities, strengthen public health and ensure people-centred health systems that are universal, equitable, sustainable and of high quality".**

Health 2020 recognizes the diversity of countries across the Region. It reaches out to many different people, within and outside of government, to provide inspiration and direction on how better to address the complex health challenges of the 21st century. The framework confirms the values of Health for All and – supported by the evidence provided in the accompanying documents – identifies two key strategic directions with four policy priority action areas. It builds on the experiences gained from previous Health for All policies to guide both Member States and the WHO Regional Office for Europe.

Health is a major societal resource and asset

Good health benefits all sectors and the whole of society – making it a valuable resource. Good health is essential for economic and social development and a vital concern to the lives of every single person, all families and communities. Poor health wastes potential, causes despair and drains resources across all sectors. Enabling people to have control over their health and its determinants strengthens communities and improves lives. Without people's active involvement, many opportunities to promote and protect their health and increase their well-being are lost.

What makes societies prosper and flourish also makes people healthy – policies that recognize this have more impact. Fair access to education, decent work, housing and income all support health. Health contributes to increased productivity, a more efficient workforce, healthier ageing, and less expenditure on sickness and social benefits and fewer lost tax revenues. The health and well-being of the population are best achieved if the whole of government works together to address the social and individual determinants of health. Good health can support economic recovery and development.

Health performance and economic performance are interlinked – improving the health sector's use of its resources is essential. The health sector is important for both its direct and indirect effects on the economy: it matters not only because of how it affects people's health and their productivity but because it is now one of the largest economic sectors in every medium- and high-income country. It is a major employer, important landowner, builder and consumer. It is also a major driver of research and innovation and a significant sector in the international competition for people, ideas and products. Its importance will continue to grow and, with it, the significance of its contribution to wider societal goals.

Across the WHO European Region as a whole, health has greatly improved in recent decades – but not everywhere and not for

everyone equally; this is unacceptable.** Many groups and areas have been left behind and, in many instances, as economies falter, health inequalities are growing within and between countries. Ethnic minorities, some migrant communities and groups such as Travellers and Roma suffer disproportionately. Shifting patterns of disease, demography and migration may affect progress in health and require improved management and governance. Rapid growth of chronic disease and mental disorders, lack of social cohesion, environmental threats and financial uncertainties make improving health even more difficult and threaten the sustainability of health and welfare systems. Creative and innovative responses, to which there is real commitment, are needed.

Rio Political Declaration on Social Determinants of Health (2011)

"Health inequities arise from the societal conditions in which people are born, grow, live, work and age, referred to as social determinants of health."

The participants declared:

"We reaffirm that health inequities within and between countries are politically, socially and economically unacceptable, as well as unfair and largely avoidable, and that the promotion of health equity is essential to sustainable development and to a better quality of life and well-being for all, which in turn can contribute to peace and security."

A strong value base: reaching the highest attainable standard of health

Health 2020 is based on the values enshrined in the WHO Constitution: "The enjoyment of the highest attainable standard of health is one of the fundamental rights of every human being". Countries across the WHO European Region have acknowledged the right to health and committed themselves to universality, solidarity and equal access as the guiding values for organizing and funding their health systems. They aim for the highest attainable level of health regardless of ethnicity, sex, age, social status or ability to pay. These values include fairness, sustainability, quality, transparency, accountability, gender equality, dignity and the right to participate in decision-making.

What is a social gradient?

The social gradient in health means that health gets progressively better as the socioeconomic position of people and/or communities improve. Thus health inequities affect everyone. This is a global phenomenon that applies to all countries, irrespective of income.

A strong social and economic case for improving health

The challenge health expenditure poses to governments is greater than ever. In many countries, the health share of government budgets is larger than ever, and health care costs have grown faster than GDP. But for at least some of these countries, data show a lack of correlation between health expenditure and health outcome. Many health systems fail to contain costs while financial pressures on them make getting the balance right for health and ensuring social protection ever harder. Costs are primarily driven by the supply side, such as new treatments and technologies, and people's rising expectations of protection from health risks and access to high-quality health care. Before being embarked on, any health reform should give careful consideration to deeply entrenched economic and political interests and social and cultural opposition. These challenges require intersectoral approaches, since health ministers cannot resolve them on their own.

Investing in health makes sense

Of the increase in health spending, 92% correlates with positive growth in gross domestic product (GDP). During the last three decades, health system spending in most countries in the Organisation for Economic Co-operation and Development (OECD) has begun to rise – on average at least 1% per year faster than real GDP across the OECD. In 1950, health spending in the United Kingdom was 3% of GDP. Even in the United States in 1970, health spending was only 7% of GDP. The average health spending in the OECD rose from 5% of GDP in 1970 to 9% in 2010.

Real health benefits can be attained at an affordable cost and within resource constraints if effective strategies are adopted. A growing body of evidence on the economics of disease prevention shows how health costs can be contained, but only if they also address inequalities across the social gradient and support the most vulnerable people. At present, governments spend only a small fraction of their health budgets on promoting health and preventing disease – about 3% in OECD countries – and many do not systematically address inequalities. Social

Prevention works …

For example, evidence from Poland shows that changes in diet and smoking reduce chronic heart disease and overall premature mortality rates.

The most cost-effective tobacco control policy is raising taxes. A 10% price increase could result in 0.6 million to 1.8 million fewer premature deaths in the countries in eastern Europe and central Asia.

… for all sectors …

The tangible benefits of increasing taxes on alcohol in England were estimated to include reductions of €183 million in health and welfare costs and €405 million in labour and productivity losses, and the cost of implementation was less than €0.10 per person (€3.7 million total).

The savings to the health service from reduced hospital admissions related to alcohol were an estimated €65 million in the first year, and €118 million of crime-related costs were saved.

In countries such as the Russian Federation, a comprehensive prevention package would cost no more than US$ 4 per person per year.

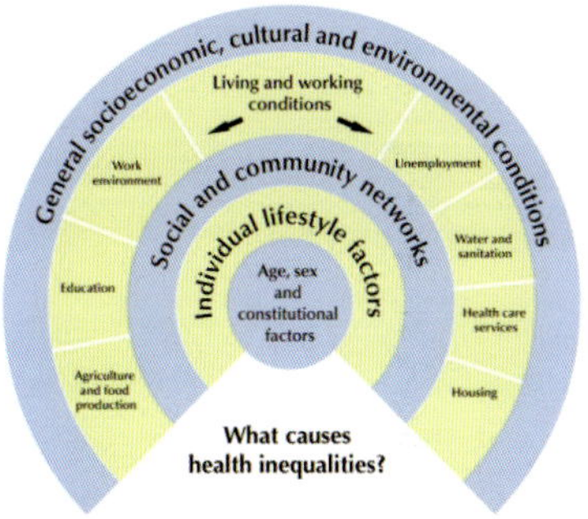

Adapted from: Dahlgren G, Whitehead M. *Tackling inequalities in health: what can we learn from what has been tried?* London, King's Fund, 1993.

… but must be targeted to reduce health inequalities

There are important inequalities within countries across key lifestyle indicators, including: smoking rates, obesity, exercise and limiting long-term illness.

In addition, the 20% of the population with the lowest income is most likely to delay seeking care because of fear of financial catastrophe from out-of-pocket payments.

and technological advances, if used effectively, offer real health benefits, especially in the areas of information, social marketing and social media.

Using resources efficiently within the health sector can contain costs. European health systems are being required to improve their performance and respond to new challenges. Reconfiguring services, acquiring new responsibilities, introducing incentives and payment structures can provide better value for money. Health systems, like other sectors, need to adapt and change. Health policy statements by such organizations as the European Union (EU) and the OECD have reinforced this.

In a globalized world, countries are increasingly required to work together to solve many key health challenges. This requires cooperation across borders. Many international agreements underline this requirement, such as the International Health Regulations, the WHO Framework Convention on Tobacco Control or the Doha Declaration on the TRIPS Agreement and Public Health (related to intellectual property).

Strategic objectives of Health 2020: stronger equity and better governance for health

Health 2020 recognizes that successful governments can achieve real improvements in health if they work across government to fulfil two linked strategic objectives:

- improving health for all and reducing health inequalities
- improving leadership and participatory governance for health.

Improving health for all and reducing health inequalities

Countries, regions and cities setting common objectives and joint investment between health and other sectors can significantly improve health and well-being. Priority areas include: preschool education, educational performance, employment and working conditions, social protection and reducing poverty. Approaches include: addressing community resilience, social inclusion and cohesion; promoting assets for well-being; mainstreaming gender and building the individual and community strengths that protect and promote health, such as individual skills and a sense of belonging. Setting targets for reducing health inequalities can help drive action and is one of the principal ways of assessing health development at all levels.

Addressing social inequalities contributes significantly to health and well-being. The causes are complex and deeply rooted across the life course, reinforcing disadvantage and vulnerability. Health 2020 highlights the increasing concern about tackling poor health within countries and across the Region as a whole. The lowest and highest life expectancies at birth in the WHO European Region differ by 16 years, with differences between the life expectancies of men and women; and maternal mortality rates are up to 43 times higher in some countries in the Region than in others. Such extreme health inequalities are also linked to health-related behaviour, including tobacco and alcohol use, diet and physical activity and mental disorders, which in turn reflect the stress and disadvantage in people's lives.

Taking action on the social and environmental determinants of health can address many inequalities effectively. Research shows that effective interventions require a policy environment that overcomes sectoral boundaries and enables integrated programmes. For example, evidence clearly indicates that integrated approaches to child well-being and early childhood development produce better and fairer outcomes in both health and education. Urban development that considers the determinants of health is crucial, and mayors and local authorities play an ever more important role in promoting health and well-being. Participation, accountability and sustainable funding mechanisms reinforce the effects of such local programmes.

Education and health together

Considerable evidence supports the claim that education and health are correlated. Data indicate that the number of years of formal schooling completed is the most important correlate of good health.

According to the 2003 *Human development report* (United Nations Development Programme): "Education, health, nutrition and water and sanitation complement each other, with investments in any one contributing to better outcomes in the others".

Improving leadership and participatory governance for health

Leadership from health ministers and public health agencies will remain vitally important to address the disease burden across the European Region. It needs to be strengthened. The health sector is responsible for: developing and implementing national and subnational health strategies; setting health goals and targets for improving health; assessing how the policies of other sectors affect health; delivering high-quality and effective health care services; and ensuring core public health functions. It also has to consider how its health policy decisions affect other sectors and stakeholders.

Health ministries and public health agencies are increasingly engaged in initiating intersectoral approaches for health and acting as health brokers and advocates. This includes highlighting both the economic, social and political benefits of good health and the adverse effects of ill health and inequalities on every sector, the whole of government and the whole of society. Exercising such a leadership role requires using diplomacy, evidence, argument and persuasion. The health sector also has a partnership role towards other sectors when strengthening health can contribute to achieving their goals. All countries at the United Nations High-level Meeting on the Prevention and Control of Non-communicable Diseases and the World Health Assembly have endorsed such collaborative approaches – referred to as whole-of-government and whole-of-society approaches.

Whole-of-government approach

Whole-of-government activities are multilevel (from local to global) government actions, also increasingly involving groups outside government. This approach requires building trust, common ethics, a cohesive culture and new skills. It stresses the need for better coordination and integration, centred on the overall societal goals for which the government stands.

In countries with federal systems or in which the regional and local levels are politically autonomous, extensive consultations across levels of government can strengthen whole-of-government approaches.

Accountability is required at all levels and in all systems.

Governments at all levels are considering establishing formal structures and processes that support coherence and intersectoral problem-solving. This can strengthen coordination and address power imbalances between sectors. The strategic benefits of adopting a health in all policies approach are increasingly being recognized. This approach advocates moving health up the policy agenda, strengthening policy dialogue on health and its determinants, and building accountability for health outcomes. Health impact assessment and economic evaluation are valuable tools in assessing the potential effects of policies and can also be used to assess how policies affect equity. Qualitative and quantitative health data can be gathered and validated to assess impact on health.

Health in all policies

Health in all policies is designed to make governance for health and well-being a priority for more than the health sector. It works in both directions, ensuring that all sectors understand and act on their responsibility for health while recognizing how health affects other sectors.

Research in well-being – as conducted in other organizations such as the OECD – can also contribute.

Governments are also committed to establishing structures and processes that enable increased involvement of a wider range of stakeholders. This is especially important for citizens, civil society organizations and other groups (such as migrants) that make up civil society. Active and committed groups are increasingly coming together to advance health at all levels of governance. Examples range from global to local levels and include: United Nations summits deliberating health; the Inter-Parliamentary Union; the WHO Healthy Cities and Communities movement; global movements to fight poverty; disease-specific advocacy such as HIV; national initiatives to define health targets; and the regional health strategies of entities such as the EU. They play a significant role in promoting health and advancing the health agenda.

Effective leadership throughout society can support better results for health. Research shows strong correlations between responsible governance, new forms of leadership and participation. In the 21st century, many individuals, sectors and organizations can provide leadership for health. This can take many forms and requires creativity and new skills, especially in managing conflicts of interest and finding new ways of tackling intractable complex problems. Together with Member States, WHO has a special responsibility to exercise such leadership and to support health ministries in achieving their goals.

Empowering people, citizens, consumers and patients is critical for improving health outcomes, health system performance and patient satisfaction. The voice of civil society, including individuals and patient organizations, youth organizations and senior citizens is essential to draw attention to health-damaging environments, lifestyles or products and to gaps in the quality and provision of health care. It is also critical for generating new ideas.

Whole-of-society approach

A whole-of-society approach goes beyond institutions: it influences and mobilizes local and global culture and media, rural and urban communities and all relevant policy sectors, such as the education system, the transport sector, the environment and even urban design, as demonstrated in the case of obesity and the global food system.

Whole-of-society approaches are a form of collaborative governance that can complement public policy. They emphasize coordination through normative values and trust-building among a wide variety of actors.

By engaging the private sector, civil society, communities and individuals, the whole-of-society approach can strengthen the resilience of communities to withstand threats to their health, security and well-being.

Contribution of civil society

Civil society is a key actor in formulating, promoting and delivering change. The WHO European Region has been at the forefront of forming innovative partnerships with civil society, including with communities of key population groups at higher risk (such as with people living with HIV) and with nongovernmental organizations that advocate for and provide services. Several pan-European networks and organizations have emerged, as the number of people living with HIV has increased.

Working together on common policy priorities for health

The Health 2020 policy is based on four priority areas for policy action:

- investing in health through a life-course approach and empowering people;
- tackling the Region's major health challenges of noncommunicable and communicable diseases;
- strengthening people-centred health systems, public health capacity and emergency preparedness, surveillance and response; and
- creating resilient communities and supportive environments.

In a spirit of coherence and consistency, the four priority areas build on the "categories for priority-setting and programmes in WHO". Those categories were agreed by Member States at the global level and have been aligned to address the special requirements and experiences of the European Region. They also build on relevant WHO strategies and action plans at regional and global levels.

The four priority areas are interlinked, interdependent and mutually supportive. For example, action on the life course and empowerment of people will help contain the epidemic of noncommunicable diseases, as will stronger public health capacity. These, in turn, will also help to contain communicable disease outbreaks. Governments achieve higher health impact when they link up policies, investments and services and focus on reducing inequalities. The WHO Regional Office for Europe will step up its role as a resource for developing policy based on evidence and examples of integrated approaches. Regional headline targets will support the monitoring of Health 2020's progress.

Addressing the four priorities requires a combination of governance approaches that promote health, equity and well-being. Smart governance will anticipate change, foster innovation and be oriented towards investing in promoting health and preventing disease. Approaches to governance will include governing through public policy and regulation as well as new forms of collaboration with civil society organizations, independent agencies and expert bodies. There is an increasing need to apply evidence to policy and practice, observe ethical boundaries, expand transparency, and strengthen accountability in such fields as privacy, risk assessment and health impact assessment.

Health 2020 recognizes that countries engage from different starting-points and have different contexts and capacity. Many health policy decisions have to be taken under conditions of uncertain and imperfect knowledge, and the wider system effects of many aspects of reforming health systems also cannot be fully predicted. Tackling complex problems such as obesity, multimorbidity and neurodegenerative diseases is challenging. Drawing on knowledge from the social, behavioural and policy sciences is proving increasingly important, including social marketing, behavioural economics and neuroscience. Studies note the value of promoting smaller-scale yet comprehensive interventions at the local and community levels, to encourage learning and adaptation. Cooperation across the European Region can accelerate the development of expertise: every country and sector can both learn and contribute.

Priority area 1. Investing in health through a life-course approach and empowering people

Supporting good health throughout the life-course leads to increasing healthy life expectancy and a longevity dividend, both of which can yield important economic, societal and individual benefits. The demographic transformation underway in countries requires an effective life-course strategy that gives priority to new approaches to promoting health and preventing disease. Improving health and health equity begins with pregnancy and early child development. Healthy children learn better, healthy adults are more productive, and healthy older people can continue to contribute actively to society. Healthy and active ageing, is a policy priority and a major research priority.

Health promotion programmes based on principles of engagement and empowerment offer real benefits. These include: creating better conditions for health, improving health literacy, supporting independent living and making the healthier choice the easier choice. Furthermore, it means making pregnancies safe; giving people a healthy start in life; promoting safety and well-being and giving protection during childhood

Health 2020 headline targets

Health 2020 strives to achieve measurable impact on health in the Region. The regional goals below have been agreed by Member States.

1. Reduce premature mortality in the European Region by 2020.
2. Increase life expectancy in the European Region.
3. Reduce inequalities in health in the European Region.
4. Enhance the well-being of the European Region population.
5. Ensure universal coverage and the right to the highest attainable level of health.
6. Set national goals and targets related to health in Member States.

A set of voluntary indicators agreed on by Member States can support national goals and targets related to health.

Health information systems support the Health 2020 process

Health information systems and services need to be developed across the Member States of the WHO European Region. The WHO Regional Office for Europe works to assist Member States in their assessment and technical improvement, and provides health information to Member States by:

- working with international partners to ensure the standardization, international comparability and quality of health data;
- working with a network of health agencies dealing with health information and evidence; and
- actively compiling, disseminating and granting easy access to health data and research evidence.

Governance for health usually requires a mix of strategies

The Moscow Declaration on Healthy Lifestyles and Noncommunicable Disease Control (2011) states:

"We ... recognize that a paradigm shift is imperative in dealing with NCD challenges, as NCDs are not only caused by biomedical factors but also caused or strongly influenced by behavioural, environmental, social and economic factors."

Evidence-informed and cost-effective strategies for reducing tobacco use have been identified, comprising the WHO Framework Convention on Tobacco Control and six MPOWER strategies supporting the Convention at the country level:

1. monitoring tobacco consumption and the effectiveness of preventive measures;
2. protecting people from exposure to tobacco smoke;
3. offering assistance for smoking cessation;
4. warning about the dangers of tobacco;
5. enforcing restrictions on tobacco advertising, promotion and sponsorship; and
6. raising taxes on tobacco.

Tobacco control interventions are the second most effective way to spend funds to improve health, after childhood immunization.

Similar evidence-informed strategies need to be developed for other systemic health risks, such as obesity. For alcohol, Member States have already adopted a global policy and a regional policy.

and for young people; promoting healthy workplaces; and supporting healthy ageing. Providing healthy food and nutrition throughout the lifespan is a priority given the obesity epidemic that is spreading across Europe.

Strong evidence indicates that cost-effective policy pathways can directly enhance population health and well-being. Practical experience and evidence on health promotion programmes and national strategies for key disease groups – such as cardiovascular disease or diabetes – have grown throughout the European Region. They demonstrate that combining government leadership, supportive environments and approaches that promote a sense of control and empowerment can lead to success. Strengthening social behavioural research can provide a growing evidence base to underpin such developments.

Strengthening mental health promotion programmes is highly relevant. One in four people in the European Region experience some type of mental health problem during their lives. A particular challenge is to promote the early diagnosis of depression and prevent suicide by initiating community-based intervention programmes. Research is leading to a better understanding of the damaging association between mental health problems and social marginalization, unemployment, homelessness and alcohol and other substance use disorders. New forms of addiction related to online virtual worlds must also be addressed.

A strategic focus on healthy living for both young and older people is particularly valuable. A broad range of stakeholders can contribute to programmes that support their health, including intergenerational activities. For young people, these can include peer-to-peer education, involvement of youth organizations and school-based health literacy programmes. Integrating work on mental and sexual health is particularly important. For older people, active and healthy ageing initiatives can benefit health and quality of life.

Priority area 2. Tackling Europe's major health challenges: noncommunicable and communicable diseases

Health 2020 focuses on a set of effective integrated strategies and interventions to address major health challenges across the Region. These are related to both noncommunicable and communicable diseases. Both types require combining determined public health action and health care system interventions. The effectiveness of these is underpinned by actions on equity, social determinants of health, empowerment and supportive environments.

A combination of approaches is required to successfully address the high burden of noncommunicable diseases in the Region. Health 2020 supports the implementation of integrated whole-of-government and whole-of-society approaches that have been agreed in other regional and global strategies, since it is increasingly recognized that action to influence individual behaviour has limited impact. Noncommunicable diseases are unequally distributed within and between countries and are closely linked to action on the social and environmental determinants of health.

Burden of noncommunicable diseases

The European Region has the highest burden of noncommunicable diseases worldwide. Two disease groups, cardiovascular diseases and cancer, cause almost three quarters of mortality in the Region, and three main disease groups, cardiovascular diseases, cancer and mental disorders, cause more than half the burden of disease (measured using disability-adjusted life-years (DALYs)). Much premature mortality is avoidable: estimates indicate that at least 80% of all heart disease, stroke and type 2 diabetes and at least one third of cancer cases are preventable. Inequality in the burden of noncommunicable diseases within and between countries demonstrates that the potential for health gain is still enormous.

Burden of mental disorders

Mental disorders are the second largest contributor to the burden of disease (measured using DALYs) in the European Region (at 19%) and the most important cause of disability. The ageing population leads to an increase of the prevalence of dementia. Common mental disorders (depression and anxiety) affect about 1 in 4 people in the community every year. However, about 50% of people with mental disorders do not receive any form of treatment. Stigma and discrimination are major reasons why people avoid seeking help.

Burden of tuberculosis

In 2010, the European Region had an estimated 420 000 new and relapsed tuberculosis (TB) cases and 61 000 deaths caused by TB. Most TB, 87% of new cases and 94% of deaths, occurs in the eastern and central parts of the Region. The Region has the lowest treatment success rate globally, reflecting the high rate of TB drug resistance; multidrug-resistant TB is found in 13% of newly treated cases and 42% of those previously treated. The disease is often linked to poor socioeconomic conditions and other determinants, including homelessness.

Health 2020 supports intensifying efforts to implement global and regional mandates in relation to noncommunicable diseases. The priority action areas for the Region include the following.

- **Existing declarations and strategies.** These include: the United Nations 2011 political declaration on noncommunicable diseases; the WHO Framework Convention on Tobacco Control; the Global Strategy on Diet, Physical Activity and Health; the global strategy to reduce the harmful use of alcohol and regional action plan to reduce the harmful use of alcohol; the action plan for the implementation of the European Strategy for the Prevention and Control of Noncommunicable Diseases 2012–2016; and the WHO Mental Health Action Plan for Europe.
- **Health promotion.** As defined in the Ottawa Charter for Health Promotion, this is at the core of these declarations and strategies. They all encourage governments to develop intersectoral national strategies with goals and targets on key challenges related to noncommunicable diseases.

Health 2020 supports continued strong efforts to combat communicable diseases. No country can afford to relax its vigilance, and each has to continually strive to maintain the highest standards. For the European Region, the priority action areas are as follows.

- **Building information and surveillance capacity:** to implement the International Health Regulations, improve information exchange and, where appropriate, implement joint surveillance and disease control activities by public health, veterinary, food and agriculture authorities to better control infectious diseases that can be transmitted from animals to humans, including emerging infectious diseases, drug-resistant organisms and waterborne and foodborne infections.
- **Tackling serious viral and bacterial threats:** to implement regional policies and action plans; to combat antimicrobial resistance; to contain the emergence and spread of drug-resistant organisms and infections through the prudent use of antibiotics and infection control; to ensure safe basic commodities such as water and food; to reach and maintain recommended immunization coverage to prevent vaccine-preventable diseases; and to reach regional and global eradication and elimination goals for polio, measles, rubella and malaria; to fully control major diseases such as tuberculosis, HIV and influenza by ensuring that the whole population, including vulnerable groups, has access to the health care system and evidence-informed interventions.

Priority area 3. Strengthening people-centred health systems, public health capacity and emergency preparedness, surveillance and response

Achieving high-quality care and improved health outcomes requires health systems that are financially viable, fit for purpose, people-centred and evidence-informed. All countries have to adapt to changing demography and patterns of disease, especially mental health challenges, chronic diseases and conditions related to ageing. This requires reorienting health care systems to give priority to disease prevention, foster continual quality improvement and integrate service delivery, ensure continuity of care, support self-care by patients and relocate care as close to home as is safe and cost-effective. The potential of personalized medicine needs to be assessed.

Health 2020 reconfirms the commitment of WHO and its Member States to ensure universal coverage, including access to high-quality and affordable care and medicines. Many countries have achieved universal coverage but much needs to be done to eliminate catastrophic and impoverishing payments in the Region. It is important to ensure long-term sustainability and resilience to economic cycles, to contain supply-driven cost increases and to eliminate wasteful spending while providing reasonable levels of financial protection. Health technology assessment and quality assurance mechanisms are especially important for health system transparency and accountability and are an integral part of a patient safety culture.

Health 2020 remains committed to a primary health care approach as a cornerstone of health systems in the 21st century. Primary health care can respond to today's needs by fostering an enabling environment for partnerships to thrive, and encouraging people to participate in new ways in their treatment and take better care of their own health. Making full use of 21st-century tools and innovations such as communications technology – digital records, telemedicine and e-health – and social media can contribute to better and more cost-effective care. Recognizing patients as a resource and as partners, and being accountable for patient outcome are important principles.

Achieving better health outcomes requires substantially strengthening public health functions and capacity. Although public health capacity and resources vary across the Region, prioritizing investment in public health institutional arrangements and capacity-building, and efforts to strengthen health protection, health promotion and disease prevention can have important cost-effective benefits. Reviewing and adapting public health laws and instruments to modernize and strengthen public health functions can also help. Cooperation on global health and health challenges of a cross-border nature is increasingly important, as is coordination within countries that have devolved and decentralized public health responsibilities.

Revitalizing public health and transforming service delivery requires reforming the education and training of health professionals. A more flexible, multi-skilled and team-oriented workforce is at the heart of a health system fit for the 21st century. This includes: team-based delivery of care; new forms of service delivery (including home care and long-term care); skills in supporting patient empowerment and self-care; and enhanced strategic planning, management, working across sectors and leadership capacity. It implies a new working culture that fosters new forms of cooperation between professionals in public health and health care, as well as between health and social services professionals and health and other sectors. The global health workforce crisis requires that the WHO Global Code of Practice for the International Recruitment of Health Personnel be implemented.

Developing adaptive policies, resilient structures and foresight to effectively anticipate and deal with public health emergencies is crucial. It is important for policies to reflect the complexities of causal pathways and respond quickly and innovatively to unpredictable events,

A health system

"Within the political and institutional framework of each country, a health system is the ensemble of all public and private organizations, institutions and resources mandated to improve or restore health. Health systems encompass both personal and population services, as well as activities to influence the policies and actions of other sectors to address the social, environmental and economic determinants of health."

–Tallinn Charter: Health Systems for Health and Wealth

Technological and scientific advances

Work on the human genome is substantially changing public health research, policies and practice, and facilitating numerous discoveries on the genomic basis of health and disease. Rapid scientific advances and new genomics tools have contributed to understanding disease mechanisms.

Nanotechnology involves manipulating properties and structures at the nanoscale. It is being used for more targeted drug therapies or smart drugs. These new drug therapies have already been shown to cause fewer side effects and be more effective than traditional therapies.

Technologies for patients and their caregivers such as self-management tools, health applications and devices to better manage their health or their chronic disease from home will contribute to changing the nature of care and reducing costs.

such as in communicable disease outbreaks. The International Health Regulations require countries to implement a multi-hazard, intersectoral and cross-border approach to public health emergencies and to be prepared to effectively manage health-related aspects of emergencies and humanitarian disasters.

Priority area 4. Creating resilient communities and supportive environments

Building resilience is a key factor in protecting and promoting health and well-being at both the individual and community levels. People's health chances are closely linked to the conditions in which they are born, grow, work and age. Systematically assessing the health effects of a rapidly changing environment – especially related to technology, work, energy production and urbanization – is essential and must be followed by action to ensure positive benefits to health. Resilient communities respond proactively to new or adverse situations, prepare for economic, social and environmental change and deal better with crisis and hardship. The WHO Healthy Cities and Communities movement provides extensive examples on how to build such resilience, particularly by involving local people and generating community ownership of health issues. Other settings-based networks provide similar experiences – such as health-promoting schools or workplaces.

Collaboration between the environmental and health sectors is crucial to protect human health from the risks of a hazardous or contaminated environment and to create health-promoting social and physical settings. Hazards in the environment are a major determinant of health; many health conditions are linked to the environment, such as exposure to air pollution and the impact of climate change, and they interact with social determinants of health.The benefits to health of a low-carbon economy and health co-benefits of environmental policies are being considered in the context of Rio +20, the United Nations Conference on Sustainable Development. Countries have begun to develop policies that benefit both the health of the planet and the health of people and recognize that collaboration between sectors is crucial to protect human health from the risks of a hazardous or contaminated environment.

Expanding interdisciplinary and intersectoral collaboration between human, environmental and animal health enhances public health effectiveness. This can include: working to fully implement multilateral environmental agreements as well as the recommendations of the European environment and health process; expeditiously expanding the scientific knowledge base; assessing the effects on health of policies in various sectors, especially those affecting both health and the environment; ensuring the continual development and adaptation of services for environment and health; and encouraging the health sector to act in an environmentally more responsible manner.

Working together: adding value through partnerships

The aims of Health 2020 will be achieved through a combination of individual and collective efforts. Success requires common purpose and broad collaborative efforts by people and organizations across society in every country: governments, nongovernmental organizations,

Public health

The WHO European Region uses the Acheson definition of public health: "the science and art of preventing disease, prolonging life and promoting health through the organized efforts of society". This is achieved through public institutions and collective action. It includes traditional services such as health situation analysis, health surveillance, health promotion, prevention, infectious disease control, environmental protection and sanitation, disaster and health emergency preparedness and response, and occupational health, among others. More recent approaches include social determinants of health, the social gradient in health and governance for health.

20 years of environment and health action in Europe

In 1989, concerned about the growing evidence of the impact of hazardous environments on human health, countries in the European Region together with the WHO Regional Office for Europe initiated the first ever environment and health process, to eliminate the most significant environmental threats to human health.

Progress towards this goal is driven by a series of ministerial conferences held every five years and coordinated by the WHO Regional Office for Europe. The conferences are unique, bringing together different sectors to shape policies and actions on environment and health in the European Region.

civil society, the private sector, science and academe, health professionals, communities – and every individual.

Key to the success of Health 2020 will be Member States and WHO working closely together and reaching out to engage other partners. Close cooperation between the WHO Regional Office for Europe, WHO headquarters and other regions lies at the core. This is supported by building wider engagement across regional networks and entities such as the Commonwealth of Independent States, the Eurasian Economic Community, the countries in south-eastern Europe and the EU.

The WHO Regional Office for Europe will fulfil its constitutional role to act as the directing and coordinating authority on international health work in the European Region. It will establish and maintain effective collaboration with many partners and provide technical assistance to countries. It will work to engage widely; increase policy coherence; contribute to shared policy platforms; share health data sets; join forces for surveillance; and support the development of new types of network- and web-based cooperation. It will act as the European Region's repository of advice and evidence on what works and will work with countries through new types of country cooperation strategies.

Working with the EU provides a strong foundation, significant opportunities and additional benefits. The 28 EU countries that comprise part of the Region have an integration and cooperation process in health based on the EU health strategy as well as policy frameworks and legal and financial mechanisms to implement them. In addition, EU candidate, potential candidate and European Neighbourhood and Partnership Instrument countries also work to progressively align their legislation and practices with EU policies. This can contribute substantially to implementing Health 2020. The joint declaration of the European Commission and WHO, which includes six roadmaps for greater collaboration, is an important step in strengthening this partnership.

Existing cooperation between WHO and international organizations active in the European Region is also being strengthened. These organizations include bodies such as United Nations agencies, the OECD, the Council of Europe, development agencies and funds and major nongovernmental organizations. Countries across the Region contribute to, and benefit from, cooperation with international organizations, and this represents a valuable resource to support the joint aims of Health 2020 and those of other sectors and organizations.

Linking with new and evolving types of partnerships for health, active at various levels of governance across the Region, will provide important support. Substantial contributions are made by innovative cooperation mechanisms such as the South-eastern Europe Health Network and the Northern Dimension policy; networks such as the WHO European Healthy Cities Network, national health cities networks and Regions for Health; subregional networks within the Commonwealth of Independent States and WHO health promotion settings networks including schools, workplaces, hospitals and prisons throughout the Region.

Working with civil society will strengthen advocacy for implementing Health 2020. Many voluntary and self-help organizations have identified health as a significant part of their remit, and many health services continue to be delivered as part of family and community care and self-care. These organizations act from the local to the global level and have

Governance for health

Governance for health promotes the joint action of health and non-health sectors, of public and private actors and of citizens for a common interest. It requires a synergistic set of policies, many of which reside in sectors other than health as well as outside of government and need to be supported by structures and mechanisms that enable collaboration.

It gives strong legitimacy to health ministers and ministries and public health agencies to reach out and to perform new roles in shaping policies that promote health and well-being.

Coherence with global health developments

Health 2020 is fully consistent with the demands and initiatives of global health development. It embodies the global vision of helping people to achieve better health included in the WHO reform process.

Contribution of WHO

WHO is in the process of reform, designed to contribute to improved health outcomes and greater coherence in global health to create itself as an organization that pursues excellence, effectiveness, efficiency, responsiveness, transparency and accountability.

Overall, the aim is to move from an Organization that delivers separate outputs through a series of technical programmes to an Organization that achieves impact, working with national authorities, through the combined and coordinated efforts of country offices, regional offices, headquarters and its outposts, all operating as part of an interdependent network.

significantly shaped the agendas for health and its social determinants. Supporting their contribution is therefore valuable for implementation at all levels.

Looking for ways to appropriately and ethically engage with the private business sector. Attitudes towards the private sector in health vary between and within countries. However, businesses are increasingly involved in every aspect of people's lives. Their influence can help to both enhance health and undermine it. Securing a stronger commitment to health from private sector actors and encouraging and rewarding their social responsibility are important goals.

Health 2020 – a common purpose and a shared responsibility

Health 2020 is an adaptable and practical policy framework. It provides a unique platform for joint learning and sharing of expertise and experience between countries. It recognizes that every country is unique and will pursue these common goals through different pathways. Countries will use different entry points and approaches but remain united in purpose. Political commitment to this process is essential, and countries have set regional targets to express this.

In an interdependent world, the need for countries to act together becomes ever more important. Today, a complex array of global and regional forces challenges people's health and its determinants. Although more people than ever before now have the chance to attain better health, no country in isolation can harness the potential of innovation and change or resolve the challenges to health and well-being.

The future prosperity of individual countries and the Region as a whole will depend on the willingness and ability to seize new opportunities to enhance the health and well-being of present and future generations. **Health 2020 supports and encourages health ministries to bring key stakeholders together in a shared effort for a healthier European Region.**

The vision for Health 2020

Our vision is for a WHO European Region in which all people are enabled and supported in achieving their full health potential and well-being and in which countries, individually and jointly, work towards reducing inequities in health in the Region and beyond.

Further information

A series of studies have been commissioned and reviewed to ensure that all analysis and action proposals in Health 2020 are well grounded in research and experience. These include the following.

- Kickbusch I, Gleicher D. *Governance for health in the 21st century.* Copenhagen, WHO Regional Office for Europe, 2012.
- *Report on social determinants of health and the health divide in the WHO European Region.* Copenhagen, WHO Regional Office for Europe (forthcoming 2013).
- McDaid D, Sassi F, Merkur S, eds. *Promoting health, preventing disease: the economic case.* Maidenhead, Open University Press (forthcoming).
- McQueen D et al., eds. *Intersectoral governance for health in all policies.* Copenhagen, WHO Regional Office for Europe, 2012.
- Bertollini R, Brassart C, Galanaki C. *Review of the commitments of WHO European Member States and the WHO Regional Office for Europe between 1990 and 2010. Analysis in the light of the Health 2020 strategy.* Copenhagen, WHO Regional Office for Europe, 2012.

Health 2020: policy framework and strategy

Contents

Foreword ... 29

Health 2020 – an introduction ... 33

Part 1. Health 2020: renewing the commitment to health and well-being – the context and drivers ... 37

Reaching out: why health is important to the whole of society and whole of government ... 38

Health 2020's underpinning values ... 41

The emerging drivers, demography and epidemiology, and the social, technological and economic case for action ... 44

Part 2. Health 2020: applying evidence-based strategies that work and the key stakeholders ... 59

Introduction ... 60

Targets ... 60

Addressing the interacting determinants of health ... 60

Improving health for all and reducing health inequalities ... 62

Building on the evidence – an integrated learning approach ... 66

Integrating new thinking from across the social behavioural sciences and strategic social marketing ... 66

Governance for health in the 21st century ... 66

Working together on common priorities for health ... 69

Investing in health through a life-course approach and empowering people ... 70

Tackling Europe's major disease burdens ... 87

Strengthening people-centred health systems, public health capacity and emergency preparedness, surveillance and response ... 105

Health security, the International Health Regulations, emergency preparedness and response to public health emergencies ... 120

Creating resilient communities and supportive environments for health ... 122

Part 3. Health 2020: enhancing effective implementation – requirements, pathways and continuous learning ... 135

Introduction ... 136

Making it happen – the challenges facing policy-makers 136
Leadership, including strengthening the roles of health ministers and the health sector 137
Developing, implementing and evaluating national and subnational health policies, strategies and plans, drawing on the contribution of various sectors 138
Adding value through partnerships and partners for health 140
Creating whole-of-society and whole-of-government responsibility for health work 142
Monitoring, evaluation and priorities for public health research 151
Health at the crossroads of challenges for the 21st century 152
A strong role for WHO 153
Looking forward 154
References 156
Annex. Glossary of working definitions and explanatory notes on concepts and terms used in Health 2020 176

Foreword

It gives me great pleasure to welcome you to Health 2020, the European health policy framework for all. Whether you are a president, prime minister, mayor, policy-maker, public health worker or community activist, Health 2020 contains information that can help you make healthier, safer and economically wiser decisions and choices.

All Member States in the WHO European Region endorsed Health 2020 in September 2012, in two forms (both of which are included in this publication). The European policy framework for supporting government and society for health and well-being provides politicians and key policy practitioners with value- and evidence-informed strategic policy advice for putting Health 2020 into practice. The longer Health 2020 policy framework and strategy provides much more detail in terms of evidence and practice related to health and well-being. It is meant especially for people who practice policy development and implementation at operational levels. It should also serve as a valuable resource for health advocates, researchers and practitioners who are looking for more in-depth information related to the various action recommendations in the shorter policy framework. Moreover, our plan is to make this longer document a living guide, providing ongoing updated links to changes in evidence and practice for everyone – in the health and other sectors – involved in developing and implementing policy.

To ensure that the best available evidence has been identified and included, the WHO Regional Office for Europe has actively worked with hundreds of public health, economic and other experts from a wide variety of academic disciplines across the WHO European Region and beyond. These experts were asked to not just describe problems but, importantly, to identify evidence about what is working and what is not working well in addressing today's health challenges in different parts of the European Region. Our focus throughout has been on ensuring that everyone experiences more equally the significant improvements in health status that have been realized across the European Region in recent decades.

Newly commissioned studies on actions to address inequities, the social determinants of health the governance approaches and the economics of disease prevention and health promotion informed the development of this evidence-informed framework. This process has made Health 2020 a unique distillate of the best public health policy evidence available.

The Health 2020 consultation involved the WHO's governing bodies in the European Region, most notably the WHO Regional Committee for Europe, whose endorsement of Health 2020 in September 2012 was a landmark for health improvement across the Region. Beyond this it also involved the Region's Member States in other ways, through their own multi-layered forms of government and through their professional and lay interests. The involvement of civil society was central to the consultation process, as was the involvement of WHO's networks, including Healthy Cities and Regions for Health. Health 2020 states clearly that today's governance for health is horizontal, dispersed and networked, and every effort has been made to involve the full richness of these influences as the development of Health 2020 was taken forward.

Our aim throughout has been to provide the scientific rationale for action: to capture and ignite the interest and involvement of everyone who will need to be engaged now and in the future. To this end, the policy framework examines both challenges and opportunities and aims to be a tool that can be used in deciding the ways forward. Too often across the Region, these opportunities are simply not being taken up, and there are even fears that the unfolding economic crisis significantly threatens our present public health gains. We continue to spend far too little on health promotion and disease prevention compared with treatment. Health 2020 argues strongly that this balance needs to change in favour of upstream interventions to prevent the later human and economic burden of end-stage disease and disability.

Key challenges and issues Health 2020 addresses include:

- new collaborative leadership approaches to bring different partners together and mobilize broad-based political and cultural support for health development;
- insights into new leadership roles and opportunities, to reach out more effectively to others within and outside government in order to arrive at joint solutions;
- ways to make an economic case for investing in health, including evidence on the benefits of and effective approaches to achieving health in all policies;
- ways to better facilitate citizen and patient empowerment as key elements for improving health outcomes, health system performance and satisfaction with health care;
- effective and efficient ways to take advantage of new networking, partnership, communication and technological opportunities;
- a common regional mechanism to build, support and maintain unity and coherence of messaging within the public health community;
- identifying gaps in knowledge and new research priorities;
- creating an ongoing communication platform for sharing the practical experiences of policy-makers and public health advocates across the Region; and
- a focus on health and well-being as barometers of development.

The Regional Office will support the adaptation of Health 2020 approaches at the national levels by:

- helping to analyse the public health situation of countries, identifying assets and needs and making recommendations for policy priorities and ways to implement and monitor impact;
- encouraging presidents and prime ministers and all other country sectors and actors to establish mechanisms for whole-of-government and whole-of-society approaches and to monitor progress; and
- supporting capacity development where needed and requested, relating to leadership, governance, engagement and communication.

Health 2020 is a WHO policy and yet a policy for everyone. It builds on a long history of global and regional policy thinking, and it is fully aligned with the WHO reform process. The Regional Office will actively promote and support its implementation in Member States. WHO alone, however, cannot succeed in making this policy framework the cornerstone of health and improving health and well-being, and will work with many partners to this end. Together we can ensure that policy-making and governance for health is better aligned with today's needs and take action to improve the health and well-being of the present and future generations.

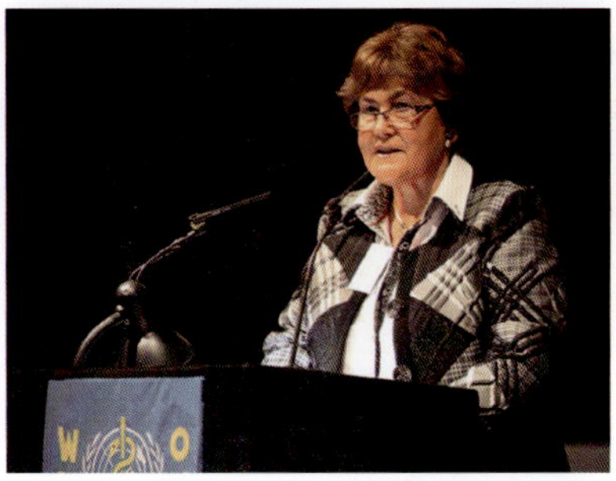

Zsuzsanna Jakab
WHO Regional Director for Europe

Health 2020 – an introduction

The 53 Member States in the WHO European Region have agreed on a new common policy framework – Health 2020.

Their shared goals are:

> … to significantly improve the health and well-being of populations, reduce health inequalities, strengthen public health and ensure sustainable people-centred health systems that are universal, equitable, sustainable and of high quality.

Health 2020 recognizes the diversity of countries across the Region

Health 2020 is intended to reach out to many different people within and outside of government, to provide inspiration and direction on how better to address the complex health challenges of the 21st century. This new policy framework and strategy identifies two key strategic directions, with four policy priority action areas. It builds on the experiences gained from the previous Health for All policies to guide both Member States and the WHO Regional Office for Europe. It accompanies *Health 2020: a European policy framework supporting action across government and society for health and well-being,* which is part of this publication.

Health is a major societal resource and asset

Good health benefits all sectors and the whole of society, making it a valuable resource. Health and well-being are essential for economic and social development and of vital concern to the lives of every person, family and community. Poor health wastes potential, causes despair and drains resources across all sectors. Enabling people to exercise control over their health and its determinants builds communities and improves their health. Without people's active involvement, many opportunities to promote and protect health are lost. This entails putting in place collaborative models of working, based on shared priorities with other sectors (such as educational outcomes, social inclusion and cohesion, gender equality, poverty reduction and community resilience and well-being). Action on those determinants of health that represent outcomes for these sectors leads to wider benefits for society and corresponding economic benefits.

What makes societies prosper and flourish can also make people healthy

Policies that recognize this fact have more impact. Fair access to education, good work, decent housing and income all support health. Health contributes to increased productivity, a more efficient workforce, healthier ageing and less expenditure on sickness and social benefits. The health and well-being of the population are best achieved if the whole of government works together to address the social and individual determinants of health. Good health can support economic recovery and development.

Health performance and economic performance are interlinked

Across the WHO European Region as a whole, health has improved greatly in recent decades – but not everywhere and not for everyone equally. Many groups and areas have been left behind and, in many instances, as economies falter, health gaps within and between countries are widening. Groups such as the Roma and some migrant communities suffer disproportionately. Shifting patterns of disease, demography and migration may severely affect progress in health and well-being if not managed well. The exponential growth of chronic disease and mental disorders, a lack of social cohesion, environmental threats and financial uncertainty make improving health even more difficult and threaten the sustainability of health and welfare systems. Determined and innovative responses are required.

A strong value base: reaching the highest attainable standard of health

Health 2020 is based on the values enshrined in the WHO Constitution: "The enjoyment of the highest attainable standard of health is one of the fundamental rights of every human being" *(1)*. Countries in the Region acknowledge the right to health and have committed themselves to universality, solidarity and equal access as the guiding values for organizing and financing their health systems. They aim for the highest attainable level of health regardless of ethnicity, sex, age, social status or ability to pay. They also include principles such as fairness and sustainability, quality, transparency and accountability, the right to participate in decision-making and dignity.

A strong social and economic case for action

The challenge that health expenditure poses to governments is greater than ever. In many countries, the health share of government budgets is significant, and health care costs have grown faster than national income. Nevertheless, data in many countries show a lack of correlation between expenditure and health outcome. Many systems fail to contain costs, while financial pressures on health and welfare systems make it ever harder to get the balance right for health. Many costs are driven by the supply side, such as new treatments and technologies, and people increasingly expect protection from health risks and access to high-quality health care. Any reform of these systems must contend with deeply entrenched economic and political interests, as well as with social and cultural opposition. Health ministers cannot resolve these challenges on their own.

Real benefits and new opportunities

Real health benefits are possible at an affordable cost and within resource constraints, if effective strategies are adopted. A growing body of evidence on the economics of disease prevention shows how health costs can be contained – but only if the measures taken also address health inequalities across the social gradient and support the most vulnerable people. At present, governments spend only a small fraction of health budgets on disease prevention – some 3% in the countries in the Organisation for Economic Co-operation and Development (OECD) – and do not systematically address inequalities. In many countries, budgets and policies in sectors other than health currently lack either a health or equity focus. On the other hand, social and technological advances provide important new opportunities to achieve health benefits – especially in information, communication and social media.

Costs can be contained by using resources efficiently within the health sector

European health systems are simultaneously being required to improve their performance and respond to new challenges. Reconfiguring services and responsibilities, redesigning incentives and payment structures, and being attentive to return on investment can result in improved value for money. Health systems, like other sectors, need to adapt and change. Health policy statements by organizations such as the European Union (EU) and OECD have reinforced this.

In a global world, countries are increasingly required to work together to solve many of their key health challenges

This requires cooperation beyond borders. Many international agreements underline this, such as the International Health Regulations, the WHO Framework Convention on Tobacco Control or the Doha declaration on intellectual property and public health.

Health as a basic human right

The right to health was first proclaimed in 1948 in the preamble of the WHO Constitution *(1)* and later the same year in Article 25 of the Universal Declaration of Human Rights *(2)*. In 1976, the International Covenant on Economic, Social and Cultural Rights *(3)* entered into force, reaffirming in its Article 12 the enjoyment of the highest attainable state of health as a human right under international law.

A level of health that leads to a socially and economically productive life

In May 1977, WHO Member States determined that the main social goal for governments and WHO should be for all citizens of the world to attain by the year 2000 "a level of health which will permit them to lead a socially and economically productive life" *(4)*. This was followed in 1978 by the Declaration of Alma-Ata on primary health care *(5)*. As part of this global movement, the Member States in WHO's European Region, at the thirtieth session of the WHO Regional Committee for Europe held in Fez, Morocco in September 1980, approved their first common health policy: the European strategy for attaining Health for All.

In May 1981, at the Thirty-fourth World Health Assembly, WHO Member States adopted this goal within the Global Strategy for Health for All *(6)*, which emphasized the attainment by societies of the highest possible level of health as a basic human right and the importance of observing ethical principles in health policy-making, health research and service provision.

In 1998, the World Health Assembly declared in its World Health Declaration *(7)* that:

> We, the Member States of the World Health Organization (WHO), reaffirm our commitment to the principle enunciated in its Constitution that the enjoyment of the highest attainable standard of health is one of the fundamental rights of

> every human being; in doing so, we affirm the dignity and worth of every person, and the equal rights, equal duties and shared responsibility of all for health.

Re-examining and renewing policy

These global and regional commitments to the right to health refer to a noble ideal. To effectively address the present challenges and seize new opportunities, the time is right for comprehensively and critically re-examining current governance mechanisms for health, health policy, public health structures and health care delivery. It is time to renew European health policy and to address the human right to health in the context of what is known and what can be achieved in promoting and maintaining health. These benefits should be available for everyone as far as possible. Achieving them will require new and radically different leadership and governance for health.

Sustainable development – linking social, environmental and economic issues and addressing inequities

A basic principle of sustainable development is that the present generation should not compromise the environment of subsequent generations. This is true for health as it is for other sectors. Social and economic inequalities, transmitted to subsequent generations, result in the indefensible persistence of health inequalities. Improving health equity, including both intergenerational inequity and the transmission of inequity, is at the core of what Health 2020 aims to achieve. Strategies for health equity and sustainable development should come together, recognizing the links between social, environmental and economic environments and intergenerational equity.

These principles are captured in the 2011 Rio Political Declaration on Social Determinants of Health *(8)*, which states:

> We reaffirm that health inequities within and between countries are politically, socially and economically unacceptable, as well as unfair and largely avoidable, and that the promotion of health equity is essential to sustainable development and to a better quality of life and well-being for all, which in turn can contribute to peace and security.

The rest of this document is organized in three parts:

- Part 1. Health 2020: renewing the commitment to health and well-being – the context and drivers;
- Part 2. Health 2020: applying evidence-based strategies that work and the key stakeholders; and
- Part 3. Health 2020: enhancing effective implementation – requirements, pathways and continuous learning.

Part 1

Health 2020:
renewing the commitment to health and well-being – the context and drivers

Reaching out: why health is important to the whole of society and whole of government

Part 1 details what Health 2020 aims to achieve, together with the current context and determinants for health and well-being and the key current social, technological and economic drivers, trends and opportunities.

Health 2020 vision, goals, strategic objectives and priorities

Health 2020 is a joint commitment by the WHO Regional Office for Europe and the 53 European Member States to a new common policy framework. The proposed vision for Health 2020 (Box 1) is consistent both with the concept of health as a human right and with a reduction in current health inequalities. Health 2020 is also consistent with existing commitments endorsed by Member States, including the United Nations Millennium Declaration *(9)* and Millennium Development Goals *(10)*, which embrace a vision of a world in which countries work in partnership for the betterment of everyone, especially the most disadvantaged people.

Box 1. The Health 2020 vision

A WHO European Region in which all people are enabled and supported in achieving their full health potential and well-being and in which countries, individually and jointly, work towards reducing inequities in health within the Region and beyond

The Health 2020 policy framework can be adopted and adapted to the different realities that make up the European Region. It describes how health and well-being can be advanced, sustained and measured through action that creates social cohesion, security, a good work–life balance, good health and good education. It reaches out to the many different actors within and outside government and provides inspiration and direction on addressing the complex health challenges of the 21st century. The framework confirms values and, based on evidence, identifies strategic directions and essential actions. It builds on the experiences gained through previous Health for All policies and guides the actions of both Member States and the Regional Office.

A vision relates to a high ideal. It needs to be translated into an achievable goal, which is expressed below (Box 2).

Box 2. Health 2020's shared goals

To significantly improve the health and well-being of populations, reduce health inequalities, strengthen public health and ensure sustainable people-centred health systems that are universal, equitable, sustainable and of high quality

Health 2020 recognizes that successful governments will achieve real improvements in health and well-being if they work across government to integrate action in two key strategic areas (Box 3).

Box 3. Health 2020's two main strategic objectives

- Improving health for all and reducing health inequalities
- Improving leadership and participatory governance for health

The Health 2020 policy framework proposes four priority areas for policy action (Box 4).

Box 4. Health 2020's four priority action areas

- Investing in health through a life-course approach and empowering people
- Tackling Europe's major health challenges of noncommunicable and communicable diseases
- Strengthening people-centred health systems, public health capacity and emergency preparedness, surveillance and response
- Creating resilient communities and supportive environments

Health and well-being – an individual state and a community resource

Health and well-being are public goods and assets for human development and of vital concern to the lives of every person, their family and community. Good health for the individual is a dynamic state of physical, mental and social well-being. It is much more than just the absence of illness or infirmity. Good health for communities is a resource and capacity that can contribute to achieving strong, dynamic and creative societies (Box 3). Health and well-being include physical, cognitive, emotional and social dimensions. They are influenced by a range of biomedical, psychological, social, economic and environmental factors that interconnect across people in differing ways and at different times across the life-course.

Health in the WHO European Region has greatly improved in recent decades. A new understanding of the determinants of health has been combined with improved knowledge of the mechanisms by which the distribution of resources and the capacity for self-determination within societies affect and create health and health inequities. The range and depth of technologies available are being transformed.

Health performance and economic performance have become interlinked. As one of the largest economic sectors in every medium- and high-income country, the health sector needs to govern its resources better. This matters not only because of how the health sector affects people's health, but also because of its contribution to the economy, within countries and internationally. It is a major employer, a huge landowner, a builder and a consumer. In these roles it reflects, and often magnifies, inequities in the wider society. The health sector is also a major force for research and innovation and increasingly a sector competing internationally for people, ideas and products. Its importance will continue to grow and, with it, its responsibility to contribute to the wider goals of society, including advocating for a positive impact on the wider determinants of health and setting an example.

Well-being

Since 1990, the United Nations has regularly measured the well-being of countries through the Human Development Index, with the intention of "[shifting] the focus of development economics from national income accounting to more people-centred policies". Starting with the *Human development report 2010 (11)*, the Human Development Index has combined three dimensions of a long and healthy life: life expectancy at birth; access to knowledge, mean years of schooling and expected years of schooling; and a decent standard of living as measured by gross national income per capita (adjusted for purchasing power parity).

The idea of generating social wealth and social growth rather than focusing merely on economic growth (measured only in terms of gross national income) has been on the international agenda for some time. Research studies in recent years have shown that unprecedented economic prosperity in the past 35 years has not necessarily made many people feel better or happier as individuals or as communities. Economic output has increased in recent decades in many countries, but levels of subjective well-being and happiness have remained flat, and inequality has increased.

Well-being itself is being increasingly studied. It is included in the 1948 WHO definition of health, although WHO has tended to focus in its reporting of health status on indicators of death, disease and infirmity, partly because information is more readily available in those domains. Today, however, policies for well-being are being considered as a possible reorientation for 21st-century public policy goals. The holistic approach of Health 2020, with its focus on healthy people and its proposals for monitoring targets for health across Europe, makes it vital to explore how well-being can be defined and measured in the context of health.

There are numerous international and national initiatives in this field, and a developing momentum of analysis, knowledge and experience. For example, the OECD Better Life Initiative addresses both well-being now (quality of life and material living conditions) and well-being in the future (sustainability). Research is ongoing in the European Union (EU) countries: COURAGE (Collaborative Research on Ageing in Europe) is a research project aiming to measure health and health-related outcomes for an ageing population. The International Well-being Group based in Australia has shown that using self-reported data about subjective well-being provides consistent outcomes, for example in the Australian Unity Well-being Index surveys. WHO is now working on contributing to this literature and experience by assembling an inventory of existing initiatives and commissioning analytical work to propose a definition of well-being, its domains, indicators and targets and options for ways of taking this work forward.

A consensus is emerging that the most important characteristics of an overarching model for measuring well-being are its multidimensional nature and the combination of objective and subjective measures. Accepting well-being as a goal for public policies requires that it be measurable. A Eurostat study has underlined that it is critical in policy-making to work with a model of well-being that covers "all aspects of well-being, including outcome measures, personal characteristics, external 'context' factors and measures of what people actually 'do' with these characteristics and 'societal' conditions" *(12)*.

Health 2020's underpinning values

Health 2020 is based on values enshrined in the WHO Constitution, namely the highest attainable standard of health and health as a human right. The Constitution expresses these values in this form:

The enjoyment of the highest attainable standard of health is one of the fundamental rights of every human being.

This is increasingly recognized as key to protecting public health and integral to a governance approach.

The specific values of Health 2020 are full recognition and application of the human right to health, solidarity, fairness and sustainability. These values incorporate several others that are important within the European Region: universality, equity, the right to participate in decision-making, dignity, autonomy, non-discrimination, transparency and accountability.

Importantly, the right to health means that governments are required to create conditions in which everyone can be as healthy as possible *(13)*. Such actions range from ensuring the availability, affordability and accessibility of health services to taking public health measures for healthy and safe working conditions, adequate housing and nutritious food and other conditions for protecting and promoting health. Citizens, in turn, need to understand the value of their health and contribute actively to creating better health in society at large.

A human–rights–based approach to health is a form of governance aimed at realizing the right to health and other health-related rights, based on responsibility by the whole of society and the whole of government. A common United Nations understanding of a human rights–based approach was agreed in 2003, and at a world summit meeting in 2005, Member States of the United Nations unanimously resolved to integrate human rights into their national policies *(14)*. Health policy-making should be guided by the standards of human rights, including eliminating all forms of discrimination and ensuring gender mainstreaming.

Governments are primarily responsible for protecting and promoting the right to health. All WHO European Member States have committed themselves in international treaties to promote, protect, respect and fulfil the right to health. In the European Region, two specific legal instruments are of particular importance for the right to health: the European Social Charter *(15)*, under the auspices of the Council of Europe, and the Charter of Fundamental Rights of the European Union *(16)*, which forms part of the Lisbon Treaty. Treaty bodies at both the international and regional levels regularly review the implementation of these state commitments. International independent experts are also appointed to monitor state compliance with health rights, such as the United Nations Special Rapporteur on the Right to Health and the Council of Europe Commissioner for Human Rights.

At the heart of human rights is the recognition that they are universal, that everybody should be treated equally and with dignity, and that all human rights are interrelated, interdependent and indivisible. A human rights–based approach to health emphasizes not only goals and outcomes but also the processes. Human rights standards and principles – such as participation, equality, non-discrimination, transparency and accountability – should be integrated into all stages of the health programming process and should guide health policy-making.

Tackling gender equality as a matter of human right and using gender mainstreaming as the main strategy for doing this are a requirement of a human rights–based approach, reinforcing the principles of non-discrimination, equality and participation. If a health care system is to respond adequately to problems caused by gender inequality, the system must be designed to address gender norms, roles and relations from the outset. Methods such as gender analysis are fundamental to realizing human rights.

Health policies and practices are based on social values. Context shapes and constructs values, both explicit and implicit ones. Further, values determine how concepts are defined, how and what evidence is generated and how policy goals are formulated and translated into practice through decision-making and action. Discussion, and even dissent, about values, either explicit or hidden, is normal in democratic political systems. Values are usually balanced against other concerns or traded off against each other. Such trade-offs are often seen in the processes of developing health policy and setting priorities, partly because health and its determinants are such complex matters, with many overlaps of interest between the government, civil society and the market. For these reasons, when the groundwork for a health policy is being laid, it is important to create clarity about the underlying values and to work through a process in which these values are promoted and upheld, both in formulating and in implementing the policy.

Societies and individuals have many goals. Interests and partners within society need to come together to achieve better health and well-being, yet health equally can and should contribute to the goals and aspirations of other sectors. The road to better health is not a one-way street, but, without health, the chances of achieving other goals in life are significantly reduced.

Health equity

Health equity is an ethical principle closely related to human rights standards; it focuses on the distribution of resources and other processes that may cause avoidable inequalities. It is a concept of social justice. Inequities in health are systematic inequalities that can be considered as unfair or unjust. Pursuing health equity means minimizing inequalities in health and in the key determinants of health.

Health inequalities that are avoidable by reasonable means are unjust – hence the term health equity to describe a social goal. Health is highly valued by individuals and society. Actions that reduce avoidable inequalities in health should be developed and prioritized. In many areas, the moral and the economic case for action come together. Investment in early child development and education may meet the demands of both efficiency and justice.

The right to health complements the concept of equity in health by implying that the reference for measuring and comparing equity should be the group in a society that has the optimal conditions for health. Health equity research and analysis are crucial for providing content to the concept of the right to health and for guiding the implementation of state obligations. Gender equity in health refers to a process of being fair to women and men, with the objective of reducing unjust and avoidable inequalities between women and men in health status, access to health services and their contribution to health.

Joint action

Where do health and well-being come from? How can these universally valued human outcomes be nurtured? We are much better able to address these questions now. Health and well-being reflect influences and interactions between individuals, populations and society stretching over time and generations. A key focus of the *European review of social determinants of health and the health divide (17)*, which extends and builds on previous analyses, is on the consequences for equity of economic, social, political and cultural processes, and how they can combine and reinforce each other to produce varying degrees of vulnerability and exclusion.

Health vulnerability results from exclusionary processes related to inequities in power, money and resources, and the opportunities of life. The review focuses on the processes – such as exclusion from good-quality education, living and working conditions – through which people become vulnerable to subsequent adversity and ill health.

These socioeconomic effects are much better understood than previously. Health experience disaggregates by socioeconomic condition, and the key determinants of the inequities in health lie in a toxic mix of poor social policies and programmes, low levels of education and unfair economic arrangements. Vulnerability results from exclusionary processes related to inequities in power, education, money and resources, and the conditions in which women and men are born, grow, live, work and age, which taken together constitute the social determinants of health. These processes operate differentially across the whole of society, create a continuum of inclusion or exclusion and give rise systematically to the social gradient in health. This gradient increases with the level of deprivation, rather than simply being linear.

That is to say, the lower a person's social position, the worse his or her health is. People in the most disadvantaged groups and communities, who are subject to many different types of exclusionary processes, experience much worse health than those subject to a single process or in a more advantaged social group. This would imply a gradient that increases with the level of deprivation, rather than being linear. Furthermore, in some societies the disadvantaged groups may be in the majority – not simply an excluded minority. Inequities accumulate over the life-course and often continue across generations, leading to persistent shortfalls in health and development potential in families and communities. Exclusionary processes produce barriers to releasing and enhancing individual and collective capabilities. When such groups as Roma,[1] migrants, people with disabilities and the very old experience multiple exclusionary processes, they become particularly vulnerable and such vulnerability becomes entrenched.

Individuals, communities and countries may have active "coping strategies" for creating sound conditions in which health and well-being can flourish. These draw on cultural resources and a wide range of positive social and environmental assets, and they should be preserved and nurtured. The focus is on resilience, on assets that protect against harm, and on reducing or altering exclusionary processes. Health assets refer to any factors (or resources) that enhance the ability to maintain and sustain health and well-being. Asset-based approaches enable and promote the protective factors that create and support health and well-being at the level of the individual, group or entire community. These factors therefore operate as a protective buffer against life's stresses and as promoting factors to maximize opportunities for health and well-being. They are linked to the control that people and communities have over their lives, and the extent to which they are empowered to exercise that control.

[1] In this publication, and in accordance with the Council of Europe's *Roma and Travellers glossary (18)*, the encompassing term "Roma" refers to various communities that self-identify as Roma and others (such as Ashkali) that resemble Roma in certain aspects but insist that they are ethnically different.

The emerging drivers, demography and epidemiology, and the social, technological and economic case for action

The emerging drivers of health: trends, opportunities and risks

Despite the real health improvements across the European Region, the challenge that health poses to governments is greater than ever. People have come to expect protection from health risks – such as unhealthy environments or products – as well as access to high-quality health care throughout the life-course. Nevertheless, the financial pressures on health and welfare systems make it ever harder to respond. In many countries, the health share of government budgets is larger than ever before, and health care costs have grown faster than gross national product (GNP). Any health reform must contend with deeply entrenched economic and political interests, as well as with social and cultural processes. Getting the balance right for health is a difficult task that health ministers cannot resolve on their own – particularly in the face of economic crisis.

The right policies and technologies can contain the upward curve of health care costs. As the health sector's share of GNP and its economic relevance increases, so does its responsibility towards others sectors and society as a whole.

While costs rise, interdependence, rapidly improving connectivity, and technological and medical innovation have all created extraordinary new opportunities to improve health and health care. The technological capacity available to understand, prevent, diagnose and treat disease has been transformed in an almost exponential progression. Diagnostic, medical and surgical interventions have expanded dramatically, as has drug-based therapy. E-health and telemedicine are examples of the transformative effects of new information technology. Nanotechnologies are on the horizon.

There is also significant new knowledge about the complex interrelationship between health and sustainable human development. Health needs to be transformed from being perceived merely as a medically dominated, money-consuming sector to a major public good bringing economic and security benefits and pursuing key social objectives. There is now a broad consensus that the health of populations is critical for social coherence and economic growth and a vital resource for human and social development.

The forces of globalization[2] are challenging all countries. Nevertheless, no country can resolve challenges to health and well-being on its own, nor can it harness the potential of innovation without extensive cooperation. Health has become a global economic and security issue. In an interdependent world, countries need to act together to ensure the health of their populations and to drive progress. These issues of managing interdependence are moving higher up the policy agenda of global policy-makers.

Policies are needed that aim to ensure decision-making power for citizens and patients, to protect their human rights, and to implement legislation that forbids discrimination. This includes securing the right to health and outlawing discrimination based on disease or disability. Shared decision-making, autonomy, independence and control over one's health and its determinants are vital. Communities are required in which people, including those with chronic diseases or disabilities, are provided with the requisite structures and

[2] Globalization has been defined as "a process that encompasses the causes, course and consequences of transnational and transcultural integration of human and non-human activities."

resources to enable them to fulfil their potential and participate fully in society. Another need is access to knowledge and to health promotion and disease prevention activities, as well as services based on respectful communication between caregivers and recipients.

All these challenges and developments exemplify the move towards a new paradigm. In addition, pressure is inexorably increasing to use health system resources more efficiently and to deliver higher quality care. There has been an important shift in the role of health professionals and citizens, with the latter now having much higher expectations in terms of information about and involvement in the services they receive. There is also the issue of medicalization to consider *(19)*, and the proper balance to be struck between societal and individual expectations and the growing capacities of the health system.

Some important new global agreements and instruments have been developed to address common health challenges, such as the Millennium Development Goals, the revised International Health Regulations and the WHO Framework Convention on Tobacco Control *(20)*. These new forms have had profound regional and national influence and more such instruments will surely follow. Other recent developments include consideration of global health in key foreign policy arenas such as the United Nations General Assembly, the group of eight industrialized countries (G8) summits and the World Trade Organization; the involvement of heads of state in health issues; and the inclusion of health issues in meetings of business leaders, such as the World Economic Forum. These developments all indicate that the political status of global health has been elevated. In 2009, the United Nations General Assembly, in its resolution A/RES/64/108 on global health and foreign policy *(21)*, reinforced this major change in perspective by urging Member States to "consider health issues in the formulation of foreign policy". In 2007, the EU launched a new strategy for public health, *Together for health: a strategic approach for the EU 2008–2013 (22)*.

Building on experience

The past three decades within the European Region have witnessed tumultuous political and social change, but "health for all" and the importance of primary health care approaches have remained as key guiding values and principles for the development of health in the Region. Health 2020 builds on that experience, detailing ways to orchestrate setting priorities around common health and well-being targets and outcomes, and catalysing action not only by health ministries but also by heads of government, as well as other sectors and stakeholders.

The comprehensive overview conducted for the WHO Regional Committee for Europe in 2005 *(23)* showed that the core values of Health for All have been broadly accepted. At the same time, it was concluded that every country had taken its own approach to developing policy and, although many countries had set targets similar to the targets for health for all, a large gap remained between formulating policies and implementing and systematically monitoring and fine-tuning them.

The Tallinn Charter: Health Systems for Health and Wealth *(24)* aimed to build on that common core set of values in 2008 and focused on the shared values of solidarity, equity and participation. It emphasized the importance of investing in health systems that offer more than health care alone and which are also committed to preventing disease, promoting health and making efforts to influence other sectors to address health concerns in their policies. In addition, health ministries should promote the inclusion of health interests and goals in all societal policies.

The demographic and epidemiological situation in the European Region today[3]

The population of the 53 countries in the WHO European Region has reached about 900 million *(26)*. Overall, health in the Region is improving, as suggested by life expectancy at birth, which reached 75 years in 2010, an increase of 5 years since 1980. Noncommunicable diseases account for the largest proportions of mortality and premature death. The four leading causes of lost disability-adjusted life-years (DALYs) in the Region are unipolar depressive disorders, ischaemic heart disease, adult-onset hearing loss, and Alzheimer and other types of dementia. Emerging and re-emerging communicable diseases, including HIV infection and tuberculosis (TB), also remain a priority area in many countries in the Region. Of special concern to all countries in the Region are global outbreaks, such as pandemic H1N1 influenza in 2009, and silent threats such as the growing antimicrobial resistance.

The determinants of health and health inequities

The determinants of health are complex and include biological, psychological, social and environmental dimensions. All the determinants interact, influencing both individual exposure to advantage or disadvantage and the vulnerability and resilience of people, groups and communities. Because these determinants are not equally distributed, this leads to the health inequities seen across the European Region: the health divide between countries and the social gradient between people, communities and areas within countries. Very importantly, many of the determinants are amenable to effective interventions. Action that takes place in sectors other than health, with the primary intention of addressing outcomes relevant to these sectors, frequently affects both the social determinants of health and health equity. Examples include education, social welfare and the environment.

Individuals, communities and countries may have capabilities and assets that can enhance and protect health, stemming from their cultural capacities, social networks and natural resources. Assets and resilience are important resources for fair and sustainable development. In drawing up its recommendations for action, the Review focuses on resilience and assets to promote empowerment and convergence of policy actions across sectors, as well as protecting against damage, reducing harm or altering exclusionary processes. Getting the balance right in the future will lie at the heart of implementing Health 2020.

Social and economic determinants

Social inequalities cause much of the disease burden in the European Region. The countries with the lowest and highest life expectancy at birth in the Region differ by 16 years, with men and women having different experiences. The countries with the lowest and highest maternal mortality in the Region differ by 42-fold. This distribution of health and life expectancy in the countries in the Region shows significant, persistent and avoidable differences in opportunities to be healthy and in the risk of illness and premature death.

Many of these differences are socially determined. Unfortunately, social inequalities in health within and between countries persist and are increasing in most cases. Extreme health inequalities also exist within countries. Health inequalities are also linked to health-related behaviour, including tobacco and alcohol use, diet and physical activity, and mental health disorders.

[3] *The European health report 2012 (25)* contains detailed information on demographic and epidemiological trends in the European Region.

With Health 2020, countries firmly commit to addressing this unacceptable disparity within the health sector and beyond. Many of these inequalities can be addressed through action on the social determinants of health.

The Commission on Social Determinants of Health *(27)* concluded that social injustice is killing people on a grand scale, demonstrating the ethical imperative of acting on these forms of inequity. Inequities in health reflect the fairness and degree of social justice in a given society and these, in turn, reflect government performance. The magnitude and pattern of social inequities in a given country result from the social, economic, political, environmental and cultural factors in that society – the social determinants of health. These are influenced to a considerable degree by policies and investment decisions, and their effects can either accrue or be ameliorated over the lives of each person. They also constitute significant losses to social and productive capital. Inequities in health are of concern in realizing the values of health as a human right and undermine the development potential of a country.

Within social systems, interactions between the four relational dimensions of power – social, political, economic and cultural – and the unequal access to power and the resources embedded in them lead to differential exposure according to, for example, sex, ethnicity, class, education and age. These differences reduce people's capacity (biological, social, mental and economic) to protect themselves from such circumstances, leading to damage to health and restricting their access to health and other services, as well as the resources essential to protect and promote health. These processes create health inequities, which feed back to increase further inequities in exposure and protective capacity and to amplify social disadvantage.

Participating in economic, social, political and cultural relationships has intrinsic value, and restricted participation adversely affects people's health and well-being. Such restriction results in other forms of deprivation: for example, being excluded from the labour market or included on disadvantaged terms, leading to low incomes, which can, in turn, lead to problems such as poor diet or housing, resulting in ill health.

Equal participation of men and women is not yet a reality in the European Region. Women are overrepresented in part-time work, have less pay for the same job and perform most of the unpaid work. In 2011, women occupied 25% of parliamentary seats, ranging from less than 10% to 45%.

These current unacceptable gaps in health experience between and within countries will increase unless urgent action is taken to control and challenge inequities in the social determinants of health.

Environmental determinants

The 21st century is characterized by many profoundly important environmental changes, requiring a broader conception of the determinants of population health. These include the large-scale loss of natural environmental capital, manifested as climate change, stratospheric ozone depletion, air pollution through its effects on ecosystems (such as loss of biodiversity, acidification of surface waters and crop effects), degradation of food-producing systems, depleted supplies of fresh water, and the spread of invasive species. These developments are beginning to impair the biosphere's long-term capacity to sustain healthy human life. The environmental burden of disease in the European Region has been estimated to be 15–20% of total deaths and 10–20% of DALYs lost, with a relatively higher burden in the eastern part of the Region.

Changing patterns of housing, transport, food production, use of energy sources and economic activity will have major effects on the patterns of noncommunicable diseases. Climate change[4] will have long-term consequences on the environment and on the interactions between people and their surroundings. This will cause a major change in the distribution and spread of communicable diseases, particularly water-, food- and vector-borne diseases.

Efforts to curb greenhouse gas emissions and other policies for mitigating climate change have significant side benefits for health. Currently accepted models show that reducing total carbon dioxide emissions in the EU from 3876 million tonnes in 2000 to 2867 million tonnes in 2030 would effectively halve the number of years of life lost from the health effects of air pollution.

Lifestyle and behavioural factors

Today, health is foremost about people and how health is lived and created in the context of their everyday lives. Health promotion is a process that enables people to improve control over their health and its determinants. Many opportunities to promote and protect health are lost without people's involvement. However, people are social actors, and supporting them in adopting and sustaining healthy behaviour requires that they be in an environment that supports that behaviour. In short, a "culture of health" is needed as one of the supportive and enabling factors for protecting and promoting the health of individual and communities. The healthy settings approach *(29)*, which has its roots in the Ottawa Charter for Health Promotion *(30)*, has been shown to be one of the most popular and effective ways of promoting environments supportive to health. It involves holistic and multidisciplinary methods and puts emphasis on organizational development, participation, empowerment and equity. A healthy setting is the place or social context in which people engage in daily activities and where environmental, organizational, and personal factors interact to affect health and well-being. Settings can normally be identified as having physical boundaries, a range of people with defined roles, and an organizational structure. Examples of settings include schools, workplaces, hospitals, markets, villages and cities.

Societal processes also influence exposure to health-damaging (and health-promoting) conditions, vulnerability and resilience. Such exposure and vulnerability are generally unequally distributed in society, according to socioeconomic position and/or other markers of social position such as ethnicity. Gender norms and values often determine exposure and vulnerability. They are also significantly influenced by a consumer society, extensive and unregulated marketing of products and, in many societies, inadequate regulation of harmful goods. The health literacy of the population has become a critical factor in enabling healthy choices and depends to a considerable degree on the skills developed from the earliest years of life *(31)*.

Today a group of four diseases and their behavioural risk factors account for most preventable disease and death in the European Region: cardiovascular diseases, cancer, diabetes and chronic respiratory diseases. Tackling issues such as smoking, diet, alcohol consumption and physical activity also means addressing their social determinants. The focus of action should be transferred upstream to the causes of these lifestyle differences (the causes of the causes), which reside in the social and economic environment.

[4] Climate change refers to a change in the mean and/or the variability of climate and its properties that persists for an extended period, typically decades or longer. The United Nations Framework Convention on Climate Change, in its Article 1, defines climate change as "a change of climate which is attributed directly or indirectly to human activity that alters the composition of the global atmosphere and which is in addition to natural climate variability observed over comparable time periods" *(28)*.

The capacity and efficiency of health systems

Finally, access to health systems and their capacity contribute to health and well-being, as well as to health care. In this sense, the health system acts as a powerful social determinant of health. This contribution can be expected to increase as technologies improve still further across the whole spectrum of health promotion, disease prevention, diagnostic and treatment technologies and rehabilitation relevant in each disease category and entity.

The role of the health system is especially relevant because of the issue of access, which incorporates differences in exposure and vulnerability and to a significant extent is socially determined. However, differences in access to health care cannot account for the social dimensions of health needs and hence only partially explain differences in outcomes *(32)*. Health systems can directly address differences in exposure and vulnerability through advocacy, by promoting intersectoral action to improve health status, and by leading by example in ensuring equitable access to care.

Health ministers and ministries have a vital role to play in shaping the functioning and contribution of health systems to improving health and well-being within society, and in engaging other sectors to address their contribution to health and its determinants. Unfortunately, their capacity to do so often falls short of what is required, and the organization of health systems has not kept pace with the changes that societies are undergoing. In particular, public health services and capacity are relatively weak, and too little attention has been paid to developing primary care, including especially health promotion and disease prevention. Further, the usual hierarchical organization of health systems makes them less capable of responding rapidly to technological innovation and to the demands and desire for participation of service users. Because of these factors, health systems are significantly less productive in producing health than they could be.

Technological developments in health care

Health technology can be defined in different ways. It can mean the procedures, equipment and processes by which health care is delivered. This would include applying new scientific areas of knowledge, such as genomics, new medical and surgical procedures, drugs, medical devices and new patient support systems. The term can also more narrowly describe the devices used to prevent, diagnose, monitor or treat diseases or conditions that affect humans. Examples would be drug-eluting stents, magnetic resonance imaging (MRI) scanners, pacemakers, minimally invasive surgery, wound and incontinence management, and devices that support self- or home management of disease, such as blood glucose testing kits, supported by counselling based on information technology.

The management of coronary artery disease provides a good example of how technology has changed the treatment and prevention of disease over time. In the 1970s, cardiac care units were introduced to manage irregular heartbeat after heart attack. Later, beta-blocker drugs were used to lower blood pressure after the attack, and then thrombolytic drugs became widely used. Coronary artery grafting became more widespread. In the 1980s, blood-thinning agents were used after heart attack to prevent reoccurrences, and angioplasty came into use after people were stable. In the 1990s, angioplasty was used more widely for immediate treatment and revascularization, along with stents to keep blood vessels open. In the 2000s, better tests were used to diagnose heart attacks, drug-eluting stents were used and new drug strategies were devised.

A well-known example of technological development is new techniques for diagnostic and treatment imaging. Techniques such as computed tomography (CT) scanning, MRI and positron emission tomography have revolutionized diagnosis and clinical practice, enabling much more accurate diagnosis in greater numbers and changing the potential and capacity of interventions.

Another example of a technological development potentially affecting practice and costs in both prevention and treatment is nanotechnology, which involves manipulating properties and structures at the nanoscale. Nanotechnology is being used for more targeted drug therapies or "smart drugs". These new drug therapies have already been shown to cause fewer side effects and be more effective than traditional therapies. In the future, nanotechnology will also aid in the formation of molecular systems that may be strikingly similar to living systems. These molecular structures could be the basis for regenerating or replacing body parts that are currently lost to infection, accident or disease. For example, nanotechnology is already being used as the basis for new, more effective drug delivery systems and is in early stage development as "scaffolding" in nerve regeneration. It is also hoped that investment in this branch of nanomedicine could lead to breakthroughs in terms of detecting, diagnosing and treating various forms of cancer.

Other examples include telemedicine, e-health (electronic health) and m-health (mobile health), which already have significant potential for increasing patient participation and empowerment and for streamlining systems of monitoring and care while reducing costs. New patient-based connectivity and medical devices allow for increasing home-based care and enable people to stay active and to contribute to society. These information technology–based developments may be linked with new self-management tools, health applications and devices for patients and their caregivers to better manage their health or chronic disease from home.

One technological development is of great potential importance. Work on the human genome during the past decade may change the nature and outcomes of disease. This work is substantially changing public health research, policies and practice, facilitating numerous discoveries on the genomic basis of health and disease. Rapid scientific advances and tools in genomics have contributed to understanding disease mechanisms. The prospect is of characterizing each person's unique clinical, genomic and environmental information, providing potential new applications for managing human health during the whole life-course. In 2005, a formal definition of public health genomics was agreed as "the responsible and effective translation of genome-based science and technologies for the benefit of human health" *(33)*. The mission of public health genomics is to integrate advances in genomics and biomedicine into public health research, policy and programmes. These advances will increasingly be integrated into strategies aiming at benefiting population health.

While there are many ethical issues to be considered *(34)*, it is likely that modern genomics will support the trend towards more personalized and individualized medicine and health care in several aspects, including health promotion, disease prevention, diagnosis and curative services. The future will see more effective tools for early detection and treatment. Developments in systems biology *(35)* should enable the progression of diseases to be detected using molecular markers, long before the first disease symptoms arise. These early markers are expected to be at the level of protein expression, as markers of the gene networks of the human genome.

All diseases have a genomic component, and host genomic factors play an important role in whether and how a disease is manifested. For some diseases (such as cystic fibrosis and Down syndrome), genetics is the only factor that makes a person sick. The disease group defined as noncommunicable diseases (including cardiovascular diseases, diabetes, obesity, osteoporosis, mental disorders, asthma and cancer) has a varying degree of genetic background, but genetics is not the only factor, as behavioural and environmental factors interact with this genetic background. This disease group is therefore also called chronic complex diseases. Even the disease group currently called communicable diseases, which used to be considered to be caused solely by infectious pathogens, is known to have a genetic component. From this perspective, the separation between communicable and noncommunicable diseases is predicted to diminish in the future and, similar to the concept of health, diseases will be approached holistically.

Various characteristics of individuals will probably be used in an integrative way for risk management, disease management and case management in noncommunicable diseases and to promote health and improve the quality of life. These characteristics include genome-based information (covering not only the genetic level but also epigenetic, expression and protein-level information); lifestyle factors, including diet, physical activity, exercise and smoking habits; mental, economic and social factors, covering home, work and social life; personal medical history and family health history; and the interaction of these factors. Another field of application where work has already started is using molecular markers to stratify diseases into subgroups to be treated with different medicines or interventions. Cancer is one of the leading fields here, with several current examples.

Securing a real paradigm shift in the use of technology depends on a willingness to restructure policies and on the ability to provide the necessary training to public health professionals. Health care systems and policy-makers urgently need to be prepared responsibly and effectively to translate genome-based knowledge and technologies into public health: this is a major task of public health genomics and an important area of potential innovation in Europe. Health policies should prepare to meet this future vision of medicine and health. This means that, instead of solely focusing on the biological determinants of health or emphasizing mainly social determinants, health will need to be approached through the perspective of all its determinants, including biological, lifestyle, environmental and social factors and the interactions between them. In the future, public health genomics will probably provide the vision and tools to integrate genome-based information (as a part of the biological determinants of health) into health care systems and policies.

Such technologically based innovations have already created new opportunities to improve health and health care. These changes substantially affect aggregate health care costs, especially when numerous organizational and professional factors support their use. This is illustrated by the dramatic increases in health care costs in the last years of life. To the extent that technology enables newer or better treatments, greater spending may involve increasing the level of health care purchased rather than unnecessary or wasted cost. Some technologies, such as the self-measurement of blood glucose, may have an upfront cost but reduce expenses related to complications further down the road.

Whether a particular new technology will increase or decrease health expenditure depends on several factors. How does it affect the cost of treating an individual person? How many times is the new technology used? On what basis can its use be rationed? Does the new technology extend existing treatments to new conditions? Does the technology cost more immediately but lead to later savings? New technologies may extend life expectancy, affecting both the type and amount of health care that people use in their lifetime. The real balance of costs and savings can often only be evaluated by long-term epidemiological and health economic studies.

The macroeconomics of health and well-being

Health – a key factor in productivity, economic development and growth

Health 2020 addresses the economic and funding aspects of health and health systems. Social progress and stability have been achieved most successfully in countries that ensure the availability of services promoting good health and education, and of effective social safety nets, through strong public services and sustainable public finances. Failure to achieve these goals can be reflected in a decline in societies' social capital of civic institutions and social networks.

Health is increasingly acknowledged as significantly affecting both the economic dimensions of a society and its social cohesion. The macroeconomics of health and well-being therefore need to be better understood. In the past 30 years, the health sector has shifted from being a functional sector focused on, and investing mainly in, health care services to constituting a major economic force in its own right. Today health is one of the world's largest and most rapidly growing industries, associated with more than 10% of the gross domestic product of most high-income countries and about 10% of their workforce. It encompasses a wide range of business sectors, services, manufacturers and suppliers, ranging from the local to the global. During the recent economic recession, the continual growth of the health care industry was a stabilizing factor in many countries. Nevertheless, its output and output efficiency clearly deserve to be maximized.

In some countries, increases in health care costs are difficult to manage and can put countries and industries at a competitive disadvantage. Health funding has therefore moved to the fore of the health debate, exploring new ways of raising revenue for health and moving away from exclusive reliance on labour-related direct taxes. These are especially relevant in social insurance systems, which traditionally use payroll taxes. As a result, the boundary between tax-funded and social insurance systems is becoming blurred, since many insurance-based systems use a mix of different revenue sources, including general taxes. These changes raise questions about effects on access to and quality of care.

The economic case for health promotion, health protection and disease prevention

Health expenditure poses a greater challenge to governments than ever before. Health expenditure has grown at a pace exceeding economic growth in many Member States, resulting in increased financial pressure that threatens the long-term sustainability of health care systems. A large burden of disease in the European Region, particularly chronic noncommunicable disease, severely affects labour markets and productivity. Diseases fuel disparities in employment opportunities and wages, affect productivity at work and increase sick leave and the demand for welfare benefits.

The development and introduction of expensive medical technologies and treatments drive up the cost of managing chronic diseases and multiple morbidities. These cost pressures provide a strong economic case for action to promote health and prevent disease. Real health benefits can be attained at an affordable cost by investing in health promotion and disease prevention. A growing body of studies on the economics of disease prevention shows how such policies can bend the cost curve of health expenditure and reduce health inequalities by focusing on the people who are most vulnerable.

Not enough use is being made of social and technological advances, especially in information and social media. These now offer huge opportunities to achieve health benefits at an affordable cost, sometimes reducing health expenditure and helping to redress health inequalities at the same time. A tangible share of the burden of disease and of the economic costs associated with it could be avoided through actions promoting health and well-being and by deploying effective preventive measures within and beyond the health care sector.

The rationale for government action to promote healthy behaviour is particularly strong in the presence of negative externalities from unhealthy behaviour or when behaviour is based on insufficient information. The victims of second-hand smoke and drunk drivers provide dramatic examples of negative externalities that can be corrected by either excise taxes on tobacco and alcohol or other policies such as public smoking bans and drink–driving laws. Inadequate consumer information justifies interventions to promote healthier behaviour by informing people about the risks of smoking, obesity and other causes of disease.

The complex nature of chronic diseases, their multiple determinants and causal pathways suggest that pervasive and sustained efforts and comprehensive strategies involving a variety of actions and actors are required to successfully prevent disease. However, the reality is that governments spend, at best, only a small fraction of their health budgets on preventing disease (about 3% of total health expenditure in OECD countries).

Expectations concerning the benefits of disease prevention must be realistic. Preventing disease can improve health and well-being, with cost–effectiveness that is as good as, or better than, that of many accepted forms of health care. However, reducing health expenditure should not be regarded as the main goal of disease prevention, because many programmes will not have this effect. Narrowing health inequalities may also be difficult to achieve through certain forms of prevention that have shown low uptake among the most vulnerable people and which therefore carry the unintended consequence of further increasing inequalities. Furthermore, the determinants of many diseases and behaviours develop through the life-course, and programmes are therefore often designed only to manage the late effects of disease.

The evidence base

The WHO Regional Office for Europe has promoted collaborative work aimed at presenting the economic case for public health action, particularly preventing chronic noncommunicable diseases. This work moves beyond what is known about the economic benefits of specific actions within health care systems, such as vaccinations and screening, to examine research endeavours to make the economic case for investing upstream – that is, before the onset of noncommunicable diseases and before health care services are required. The work highlights priority actions supported by sound cost–effectiveness or cost–benefit analyses, including actions to limit risky behaviour such as tobacco use and alcohol consumption, to promote physical and mental health through diet and exercise, to prevent mental disorders and to decrease preventable injuries, such as from road crashes, and exposure to environmental hazards. The full results of this work are forthcoming *(36)*, but some of the early evidence is presented below.

Strong evidence indicates the cost–effectiveness of tobacco control programmes, many of which are inexpensive to implement and have cost-saving effects. Such programmes include raising taxes in a coordinated way with a high minimum tax (the single most cost-effective action), encouraging smoke-free environments, banning advertising and promotion, and deploying media campaigns. Adequate implementation and monitoring, government policies independent of the tobacco industry and action against corruption are all needed to support effective policies.

A substantive evidence base of systematic reviews and meta-analyses supports the cost–effectiveness of alcohol policies. Impressive cost-effective interventions include restricting access to retailed alcohol; enforcing bans on alcohol advertising, including in social media; raising taxes on alcohol; and instituting a minimum price per gram of alcohol. Less, but still cost-effective measures include enforcing drink–driving laws through breath-testing; delivering brief advice for higher-risk drinking; and providing treatment for alcohol-related disorders.

Actions to promote healthy eating are especially cost-effective when carried out at the population level. Reformulating processed food to decrease salt, *trans*-fatty acids and saturated fat is a low-cost intervention that may be pursued through multistakeholder agreements, which may be voluntary or ultimately enforced through regulation. Fiscal measures (including taxes and subsidies) and regulating food advertising for children also have a low cost and a favourable cost–effectiveness. However, conflicting interests could hinder feasibility. Programmes to increase awareness and information, such as mass-media campaigns and food labelling schemes, are efficient investments but have poorer effectiveness, particularly in lower socioeconomic groups.

Promoting physical activity through mass-media campaigns is a very cost-effective action and relatively inexpensive. However, returns in terms of health outcomes may be lower than those provided by more targeted interventions, for instance at the workplace. Changes in the transport system and the wider environment have the potential to increase physical activity, but they require careful evaluation to ascertain their affordability and feasibility, and whether the changes reach those with greater health and social needs. Actions targeting the adult population and individuals at higher risk tend to produce larger effects in a shorter time frame.

Robust evidence indicates that preventing depression, the single leading cause of disability worldwide, is feasible and cost-effective. Depression is associated with premature death and reduced family functioning, it directly affects people's individual behaviour and it entails extremely high economic costs due to health care and productivity losses, which can be partly avoided through appropriate forms of prevention and early detection. Evidence supports actions across the life-course, starting with early action in childhood to strengthen social and emotional learning, coping skills and improved bonds between parents and children, which can generate benefits lasting into adulthood.

Sound economic evidence supports action to prevent road crashes, such as modifying road design, one-way streets, urban traffic-calming (including mandatory speed limits enforced by using physical measures), and camera and radar speed enforcement programmes, especially in higher-risk areas. Actively enforcing legislation to promote good road safety behaviour can also be highly cost-effective.

Evidence from economic studies supports action to tackle environmental chemical hazards. Examples include comprehensive regulatory reform such as that implemented in 2007 under the European Community regulation on the registration, evaluation, authorization and restriction of chemicals (REACH); the removal of lead-based paint hazards; the abatement of mercury pollution from coal-fired power plants; and the abatement of vehicle emissions in high-traffic areas, such as through the congestion charging schemes used in many metropolitan areas, which may produce savings in health care and other costs associated with childhood asthma, bronchiolitis and other respiratory illnesses in early life.

Investing in education is also investing in health. A growing body of empirical research suggests that, when countries adopt policies to improve education, the investment also pays off in terms of healthier behaviour and longer and healthier lives. For example, studies of compulsory schooling reforms adopted in several countries in the European Region conclude not only that the reforms lead to additional years of completed schooling but also that the additional schooling reduces the population rates of smoking and obesity. When countries consider the return on investment in education and other social determinants of health, the analysis should include the potential health gains.

Key approaches

Chronic diseases can be tackled cost-effectively through interventions aimed at modifying behavioural and lifestyle risk factors. This is likely to reduce health inequalities within countries in the long term. However, turning the tide of diseases that assumed epidemic proportions during the twentieth century requires fundamentally changing the social norms that regulate individual and collective behaviour. Such changes require wide-ranging prevention strategies addressing multiple determinants of health across social groups.

Most countries are striving to improve health education and information. However, solely providing information is rarely effective (or cost-effective) in influencing behaviour, and in some instances it can increase inequalities. Instead, adopting a wider strategic whole-systems approach is essential to increase the impact and effectiveness of efforts. Strategies are needed to directly address the factors within a person's own control, empowering people and ensuring a clear strategic focus on the individual or community behavioural determinants. Furthermore, the factors that may lie outside their immediate control ensure a clear strategic focus on the wider social determinants that strongly influence individual behaviour. More stringent measures, such as regulating advertising or fiscal measures, are more intrusive on individual choices and more likely to generate conflict among relevant stakeholders, but they are also likely to weigh less on public finances and to produce health returns more promptly.

Changing the behaviour of the population and fostering healthy lifestyles is challenging, but increasing evidence about what works clearly supports adopting strategic and multifaceted approaches to strengthening capability through greater control and empowerment. Although the conventional approach is to attempt to raise awareness through communication campaigns, the evidence indicates that simply providing information about unhealthy and healthy behaviour is not effective in achieving and sustaining behaviour. Health communication and education initiatives should be delivered as part of a wider portfolio of interventions aimed at creating a social and physical environment that fosters healthy behaviour. The various behavioural strategies are mutually reinforcing, and the effectiveness of behavioural programmes and interventions increases when they are integrated alongside additional strategies that address the wider social determinants.

A wide range of regulatory and fiscal measures have increasingly been put in place in many countries, for instance to the curb consumption of tobacco and alcohol. A minimum age has been set for purchasing cigarettes and alcoholic drinks, which often carry health warnings printed on their labels. Advertising has been severely restricted, and high taxes have been imposed on the consumption of both commodities. All these measures have contributed to containing consumption, and WHO work has shown that most have very favourable cost–effectiveness profiles. However, fiscal measures are complex to design and enforce; their impact may be unpredictable; and they can bear more heavily on people with low incomes than on those with higher incomes.

The recent economic crisis

Health 2020 is a policy framework that is fit for both good and less good economic times. Nevertheless, lessons can be learned from the recent economic downturn and financial crisis. The health and social sectors are especially vulnerable to cuts during economic downturns, not only because of their size within any government's budget but also because of the often relatively weak negotiating position of health ministries. In the Tallinn Charter (24), Member States declared that "today, it is unacceptable that people become poor as a result of ill health", but this can be undermined as governments look to shift the burden of financing to households as a policy response to fiscal pressures. The economic crisis presents a great challenge for Member States in how to remain committed to equity, solidarity and financial protection, but it also presents an opportunity to advocate for and invest in health and to strengthen health systems.

The recent economic crisis has affected many countries in the European Region and challenged commitments to social welfare objectives, including health and equity, which need to be reinforced during economic downturns so that the policy responses to address the economic crisis reflect public priorities rather than short-term needs to balance the budget by across-the-board cuts. Indeed, lessons from previous economic shocks experienced by countries in the Region offer insights to today's policy-makers on how to mitigate adverse effects on health and welfare of the population: health systems with strong leadership and well-functioning governance arrangements perform better in general, and especially during a crisis.

The health effects of economic crises are complex, and new evidence continues to emerge. Road traffic accidents and obesity may be reduced with declining incomes and higher prices, and social cohesion may increase. Nevertheless, psychosocial stress increases during times of economic hardship, leading to more suicides, a range of unhealthy types of behaviour and greater demand for health services for both physical and mental health needs.

Although the balance of evidence needs to be further examined, health systems must continue to function during times of economic downturn and to step up activities related to psychosocial support, particularly for poor and vulnerable people, in order to prevent severe effects on health outcomes. Beyond health effects, budget cuts lead to an increased financial burden on people seeking care in general and medicines in particular. Shifting a significant financial burden from pooled public sources to individuals receiving care via increased direct payments (user fees and co-payments) may put households at greater risk of impoverishment from ill health and reduce the utilization of health services. This may eventually result in higher costs to the health system and worse health outcomes for individuals.

Social welfare spending has major effects on health. Evidence indicates that a rise in such spending is associated with a sevenfold greater reduction in mortality than a rise of similar magnitude in gross domestic product *(37)*. In countries that have maintained, or even increased, social welfare spending when public expenditure on health was being drastically reduced, the impoverishing effects of the cuts were very small.

The WHO Regional Office for Europe and the Government of Norway jointly convened a high-level meeting in 2009 in Oslo. Recommendations were put forward for guiding pro-health and pro-poor policy responses, such as giving priority to cost-effective public health and primary health care services. Participants also recognized the importance of ensuring the efficient use of public funds (more health for the money), which is a prerequisite to effective advocacy for more money for health. The Oslo recommendations argue for introducing new taxation on sugar and salt consumption, as well as increased levies on alcohol and tobacco, fiscal measures that are concurrently effective public health interventions.

Member States have employed a range of actions to continue striving for improving health and protecting populations from the financial hardship associated with seeking care. These instruments can be grouped as follows.

- *Thinking long-term.* One option is to implement counter-cyclical public financing by accumulating reserves in health insurance funds ("save in good times to spend in bad times") or to reallocate tax revenues for health during recession. These countercyclical policies can provide a buffer in the short run and potentially prevent countries from taking drastic measures with adverse effects on the health of the population.
- *Avoiding across-the-board budget cuts.* If budgets need to be reduced for fiscal reasons, it is important not to do this in an across-the-board manner but rather in a targeted manner driven by objectives. A widely used and relatively safe option is to delay investment, which may allow the health sector to maintain the level and volume of health services, including public health services, provided that infrastructure has been properly maintained prior to the crisis.
- *Targeting public expenditure better according to social need and so protecting poor and vulnerable people.* Maintaining access to health services by poor and vulnerable people may reduce the dramatic consequences of a severe economic downturn. Changing the range of services included in the statutory benefits package can be a valuable tool for setting priorities in the health system, particularly if changes are based on evidence and aim to promote the use of high-value (cost-effective) care and discourage the use of low-value care.
- *Seeking efficiency gains by using medicines and technologies more wisely.* For all countries, an important option for mitigating the effect of the crisis is to improve the efficiency with which services are delivered to the population. Several countries achieved efficiency gains, for example, through more cost-effective use of medicines and by applying health technology assessment to inform reimbursement decisions. Some also introduced cost-containment measures by announcing overall price cuts for manufacturers and negotiating lower prices, more efficient purchasing of medicines through tendering, enhancing policies on prescribing and using generic medicines, reducing distribution margins for wholesalers and pharmacies, and taking measures to increase the rational prescribing of medicines.
- *Seeking efficiency gains by rationalizing service delivery structures.* When the level of funding to health care providers, and in particular to hospitals, is reduced, providers may themselves engage in rationing, for example by delaying, denying and diluting clinical services ("quality skimping"), unless difficult structural decisions are taken to improve the efficiency of

the hospital sector. The crisis provides an opportunity to introduce long overdue efficiency-enhancing reforms that may have been politically less feasible before the crisis. Savings are hard to realize in the short run, and the risk of failure to provide people with proper health care during the transition is high, but with careful implementation the long-term benefits are substantial.

Health ministries and governments have an important leadership role to play in general. Although preventing economic downturns may not be possible, governments can prepare better for the challenges they will face. Attention to efficiency and responsible management of public resources in the health sector, combined with prudent fiscal policy in the public sector as a whole, is essential during the years of economic growth, because in times of economic crisis the population may be more likely to need social and health services, for which sufficient public funding is required to ensure equity and efficiency in providing universal coverage. The countries that entered the economic downturn with the ability to use reserves or sustain deficit spending have been much better able to protect their populations from the consequences of the crisis. Navigating through the crisis is truly a whole-of-government responsibility.

"Wicked" problems and systems thinking

Today's health problems are difficult to solve because of their complexity, multifaceted and multilevelled nature, and rapidly changing dynamics. Economic, social political and cultural processes operate throughout life, determining social position and cohesion. Problems such as obesity, alcohol misuse, narcotic drug use, increasing health inequities, demographic shifts, environmental threats, major disease outbreaks, financial pressures on health and welfare system, and social and technological transformations all increase the need for policy innovation. The term "wicked" problems *(38)* has been applied to such issues that are difficult to solve because of their incomplete, unstable, contradictory and changing features. Many 21st-century health challenges are wicked problems. Attribution is complex, and linear relationships between cause and effect are hard to define. Wicked problems need to be considered and analysed as complex open systems.

Given these challenges, policies should be implemented as large-scale experiments in which monitoring and evaluation efforts provide an essential mechanism for the policy community to learn from the experiences acquired in practice and to adapt accordingly. Obesity is an excellent example of a 21st-century wicked health challenge. The risk patterns and behaviour associated with the spread of the obesity epidemic are complex and multidimensional. Risks are local (such as the absence of playgrounds or lack of bicycle lanes), national (such as the lack of food labelling requirements) and global (trade and agriculture policies). Only a systems-wide approach and multiple interventions at different levels of governance, which recognize the complexity and wicked nature of tackling obesity, will stand any chance of success *(39)*.

Part 2

Health 2020: applying evidence-based strategies that work and the key stakeholders

Introduction

Part 2 of Health 2020 starts with a set of targets that apply to the whole of the WHO European Region and which capture the essence of the policy framework. It then details evidence-based strategies that work for different entry points and actors. Part 2 is structured around the two main strategic objectives of the policy – improving health for all and reducing health inequalities, and improving leadership and participatory governance for health – and the four common areas for policy action. These are: investing in health through a life-course approach and empowering people; tackling Europe's major health challenges of noncommunicable and communicable diseases; strengthening people-centred health systems, public health capacity and emergency preparedness, surveillance and response; and creating resilient communities and supportive environments. Common priority areas are described. Change is essential – the new reality requires policy action necessitating that health ministries involve other sectors.

Targets

Health 2020 includes headline, overarching regional targets that will be supported by appropriate indicators and reported as regional averages. It is intended that these targets will be both quantitative and qualitative where appropriate and "smart": (specific, measurable, achievable, relevant and time-bound). Each will represent real potential progress across the processes, outputs and outcomes of the Health 2020 policy framework.

The targets are elaborated in three main areas, which support the two strategic objectives and four policy priorities that underpin Health 2020, as illustrated in Box 5 below. These three main areas are:

- burden of disease and risk factors
- healthy people, well-being and determinants
- processes, governance and health systems.

The use of targets is not an end in itself. Targets promote health and well-being by improving performance and accountability. These targets are regional in the sense that they are agreed and will be monitored at the regional level. Depending on their circumstances, all Member States will contribute to the achievement of these targets and will monitor progress accordingly. Each Member State will decide the pattern and pace of implementation and is encouraged to set national goals and targets related to health. The targets have been developed in such a way that routinely collected health information may be used to a maximum extent and new data collection avoided. Box 5 shows the regional targets for Health 2020.

Addressing the interacting determinants of health

Health 2020 as a whole highlights the very real health challenges that countries face across the Region. Although the pattern in each country may vary, the key overarching issues increasingly apply to all. However, Health 2020 goes beyond merely describing the issues; it focuses on potential solutions and areas where the evidence suggests that positive action can have important effects. In doing so, it provides an underpinning framework based on the

Box 5. Regional targets for Health 2020			
Health 2020 broad target area	**Target**	**Link with Health 2020 strategic objective**	**Link with Health 2020 policy priority**
1. Burden of disease and risk factors	1. Reduce premature mortality in Europe by 2020	1. Improving health for all and reducing the health divide	2. Tackling Europe's major health challenges of noncommunicable and communicable diseases
2. Healthy people, well-being and determinants	2. Increase life expectancy in Europe	1. Improving health for all and reducing the health divide	1. Investing in health through a life-course approach and empowering people 4. Creating resilient communities and supportive environments
	3. Reduce inequities in health in Europe (social determinants target)	1. Improving health for all and reducing the health divide	1. Investing in health through a life-course approach and empowering people 4. Creating resilient communities and supportive environments
	4. Enhance well-being of the European population	1. Improving health for all and reducing the health divide	1. Investing in health through a life-course approach and empowering people 4. Creating resilient communities and supportive environments
3. Processes, governance and health systems	5. Universal coverage and the "right to health"	2. Improving leadership and participatory governance for health	3. Strengthening people-centred health systems, public health capacity and emergency preparedness
	6. Member States set national targets	2. Improving leadership and participatory governance for health	3. Strengthening people-centred health systems, public health capacity and emergency preparedness

importance of adopting strategic approaches that assess challenges from a whole-system perspective.

It does this by recognizing that the various determinants of health are interrelated, with a mix of biophysical, psychological, social and environment factors all being important. This reinforces the importance of developing multifaceted strategies that avoid a one-off or isolated campaigns approach and instead seek to mobilize action across a range of areas to achieve a combined synergistic effect on the challenges being addressed.

The classic and well-known model shown below (Fig. 1) helps to illustrate the interrelationships between the different determinants of health, recognizing that it is important to consider both the factors that directly influence individual and community behaviour and the important wider social determinants. The social determinants are especially important to address because not only can they directly influence health (such as the effects of poor housing or sanitation) but, importantly, they also influence the genuine options and choices people have, their life chances and circumstances, which in turn affect their personal decisions and choices and lifestyles.

Improving health for all and reducing health inequalities

The Commission on Social Determinants of Health *(27)* set out three main principles for action.

- Improve the conditions of daily life – the circumstances in which people are born, grow, live, work and age.
- Tackle the inequitable distribution of power, money and resources – the structural drivers of the conditions of daily life – globally, nationally and locally.
- Measure the problem, evaluate action, expand the knowledge base, develop a workforce that is trained in the social determinants of health and raise public awareness about the social determinants of health.

Addressing political, social, economic and institutional environments is vital for advancing the health of the population. Intersectoral policies are both necessary and indispensable. Whole-of-government responsibility for health requires that the entire government at all levels of responsibility fundamentally considers effects on health in developing all regulatory and social and economic policies *(41)*.

Health and well-being can be significantly improved when countries, regions and cities set common objectives and carry out joint investment by health and other sectors. Priority areas include educational performance, employment and working conditions, social protection and reducing poverty. Approaches include addressing community resilience, social inclusion and cohesion and promoting assets for well-being, that is, the individual and community strengths that protect and promote health, such as individual skills and a sense of belonging. Setting year-on-year targets or reducing health inequalities can help drive action, as one of the main ways of assessing health development at all levels. Action must be both systematic and sustained.

Addressing social inequalities contributes substantially to health and well-being. Reducing health gradients requires a comprehensive policy goal of equalizing health chances across socioeconomic groups, including remedying

Fig. 1. The interacting determinants of health

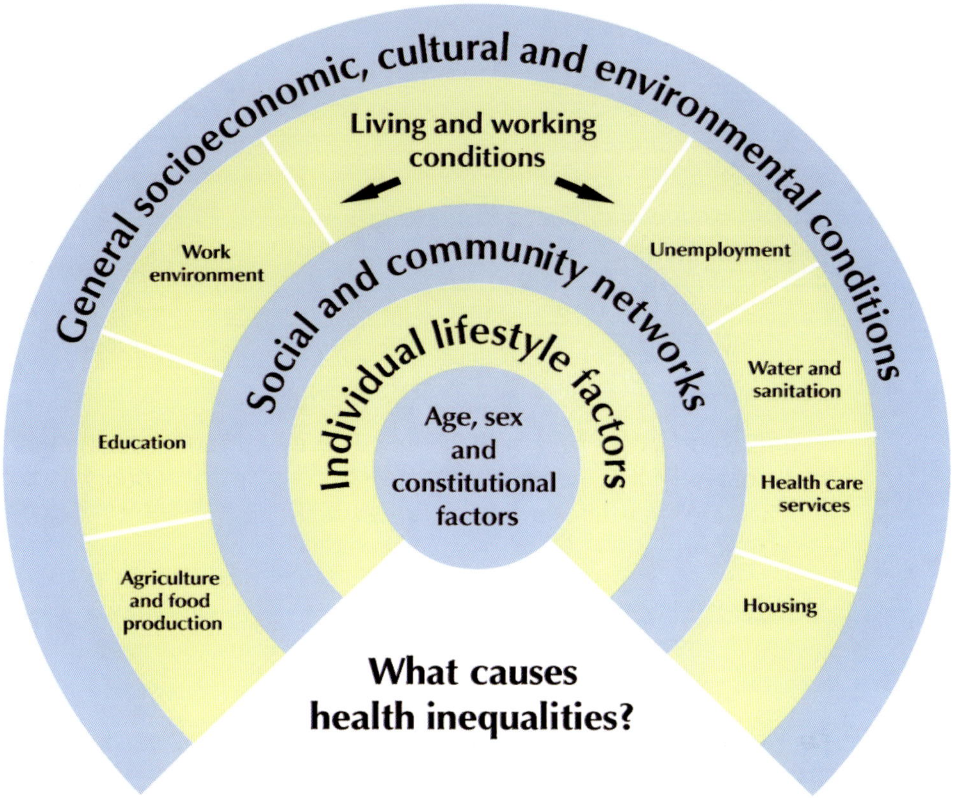

Adapted from Dahlgren & Whitehead *(40)*.

health disadvantage and narrowing health gaps. Action to reduce these inequities will touch all those affected if it is applied universally across society. Universal social protection will reduce poverty and have greater effects on people in need than narrowly targeted programmes. Nevertheless, inequity will only be reduced cost-effectively if the intensity of the action taken is proportionate to the needs of each individual or group in society. In this context, needs means the health and social problems that are amenable to action by reasonable means that are known to be effective. With this approach, action is greatest in addressing the needs of the most deprived and vulnerable people but is not delivered exclusively to them.

Taking action on the social and environmental determinants of health can effectively address many types of inequalities in health. Inequities in health cannot be reduced without addressing inequities in the causes of ill health – the conditions of daily life and the distribution of power, money and resources. These are reflected, for example, in gender and other social inequities, unequal exposure to harm and differential levels of resilience and unfairness in the immediate, visible circumstances of people's lives – their access to health care, schools and education, their conditions of work and leisure, their homes, communities, towns and cities – and their chances of leading a flourishing, healthy life *(8,27,42,43)*. Addressing these inequities means that everyone should have a minimum standard of healthy living, based on the material conditions that ensure a decent life and a good start in life (universal access to high-quality early-years development, education and employment); and empowerment – that is control over one's life, a political voice and the ability to participate in decision-making processes. Fully realizing these human rights is critical for improving health and reducing inequity, and Member States have an obligation to respect, protect and fulfil them *(27,44,45)*.

Action should be taken on a universal basis but, given the social gradient in health, delivered with an intensity that relates to social and health needs – proportionate universalism *(46)*. Reducing the socioeconomic gradient and the overall health gap within a given population requires that health improve at a faster rate in the lowest socioeconomic groups than in the highest ones. Accordingly, addressing the social gradient requires efforts not only targeting the most vulnerable people. The gradient approach implies a combination of broad universal measures with strategies targeted at high-risk groups. An approach targeting only disadvantaged groups would not alter the distribution of the determinants of health across the whole socioeconomic spectrum.

A statement of the action that is needed globally was summarized in the World Health Assembly's 2009 resolution WHA62.14 on reducing health inequities through action on the social determinants of health *(47)*. The recent World Conference on Social Determinants of Health held in Rio de Janeiro, Brazil also adopted a statement of the action needed globally *(8)*, yet real change will require more than declarations alone, even when they are backed by powerful evidence and good will. As follow-up to the World Health Assembly resolution and the Conference, a WHO strategy and global plan of action on the social determinants of health (2012–2017) is now being elaborated. Addressing socially determined inequities in health requires strong political commitment, integrated action, a strong systems approach, effective and high-performing systems and policy coherence across a range of government policies, particularly, but not exclusively, health *(48,49)*.

Taking an approach based on the social determinants of health is often contrasted with one based on opportunities, free will and personal responsibility for health, for example for health-determining behaviour. In practice, however, since analysis of high mortality rates (outcomes) shows that these result from the conditions in which people are born, grow, live, work and age, it is plainly difficult for individuals to take personal responsibility for their health without social action to create the conditions in which people can have control over their lives. In practice, the debate is not about whether reducing inequity in health outcomes is desirable but about what is avoidable by reasonable means *(50)*. To be effective, the measures adopted need to command public and political support.

It is recommended that all 53 countries in the European Region establish clear strategies to redress the current patterns and magnitude of health inequities by taking strong action on the social determinants of health (Box 6), as part of a whole-system strategic approach, that balances measures focusing on individual and community behavioural factors. It is recognized that countries are at very different starting points in terms of health, health equity, and social and economic development. While this may limit what is feasible in the short term and the timescale for addressing specific issues, it should not affect the long-term aspirations of the strategy.

Box 6. Areas to be covered by strategies for reducing health inequities

The areas covered by the strategies should include the following.

Life-course stage

Ensure adequate social and health protection for women, mothers-to-be and young families.

Provide universal high-quality and affordable early-years education and care system.

Eradicate exposure to unhealthy, unsafe work and strengthen measures to secure healthy workplaces and access to employment and high-quality work.

Take coherent effective intersectoral action to tackle inequalities at older ages, both to prevent and manage the development of chronic morbidity and to improve survival across the social gradient.

Wider society

Improve the level and distribution of social protection, according to need, in order to improve health and address health inequalities.

Mobilize and ensure concerted efforts to reduce inequalities in the local determinants of health, through both co-creation and partnership with those affected, civil society and a range of civic partners.

Take action on socially excluded groups, building on and extending systems already in place for the wider society, with the aim of creating systems that are more sustainable, cohesive and inclusive.

Adopt a gender equity approach in order to understand and tackle socioeconomic and health inequities between men and women.

Broader context

Use the system of taxes and transfers to promote equity. The proportion of the budget spent on health and social protection programmes should be increased for countries below the current EU average.

Plan for the long term and safeguard the interests of future generations by identifying links between environmental, social and economic factors and all policies and practices.

Systems

Governance for the social determinants of health and health equity requires greater coherence of action across all sectors (policies, investment and services) and stakeholders (public, private and voluntary) at all levels of government (transnational, national, regional and local).

The long-term nature of equitably preventing and treating ill health requires a comprehensive response, in order to achieve sustained and equitable change in preventing and treating ill health.

There should be regular reporting and public scrutiny of inequalities in health and their social determinants at all levels of governance, including at transnational, national, regional and local levels.

Building on the evidence – an integrated learning approach

Although the challenges are significant, there is a growing body of evidence about what works to improve individuals' and communities' health and well-being. With so many different influences on health, this means that understanding of, and insights into, what works is spread in practice across a diverse range of academic and professional disciplines. In the health sector in particular, approaches and learning are often strongly informed by a biophysical and medical sciences perspective. Although this is clearly of huge importance, it is limiting and unidimensional in isolation. As a result, there has been a growing appreciation of the need to better integrate learning from other sectors, especially contributions from the wide range of social and behavioural sciences.

Integrating new thinking from across the social behavioural sciences and strategic social marketing

Understanding of the factors that influence human behaviour has developed significantly in recent years. This has highlighted the fact that old-style message communication approaches, focused on crafting information and sending messages, are rarely enough on their own to positively affect people's health behaviour and choices. Instead, integrated learning from across the wider social behavioural sciences, including strategic social marketing, social psychology, behavioural economics and neuroscience, are increasingly providing practical and often cost-effective solutions to addressing the diversity of behavioural challenges in various populations. Moving beyond communication to a stronger behavioural focus and understanding in health and related programmes offers growing potential to achieve measurable and sustained effects in people's lives, by finding ways to practically support them in realizing their own health goals. This, coupled with a strategic focus on the wider social determinants of health, is helping to strengthen the robustness and effectiveness of interventions.

Governance for health in the 21st century

Improving leadership and participatory governance for health

Leadership from health ministers and public health agencies will remain vitally important to address the health burden across the European Region and needs to be strengthened. This leadership role for health highlights both the economic, social and political benefits of good health and the adverse effects of ill health and inequities in health and its determinants on every sector, the whole of government and the whole of society. Here health ministers and ministries and public health agencies need to take on new roles in shaping policies that promote health and well-being, by reaching out and promoting policies that benefit health for all in all partnerships beyond the health sector. Exercising this leadership role requires using a range of skills and competencies, including diplomacy, evidence, argument and persuasion.

Nevertheless, new forms of governance for health are also required throughout society and government. Governance may be variously defined. The following definition is used in Health 2020: "the attempts of governments or other actors to steer communities, whole countries or even groups of countries in the pursuit of health as integral to well-being through both whole-of-government and whole-of-society approaches" *(51)*. This definition positions health and well-being as key features of what constitutes a successful and well-performing society in the 21st century. Making whole-of-society and whole-of-government responsibility for health work and become a reality also requires strong leadership. Policy, action and a social commitment to health will not happen by themselves. The influences on health are so diverse and diffuse in modern societies that promoting and advancing health requires action based on this new thinking and a new paradigm: traditional linear, rational planning models will no longer suffice.

There has been an ongoing transformation of governance from a state-centred to a collaborative model in which governance is produced collectively between a wide range of state and societal actors, including ministries, parliaments, agencies, authorities, commissions, businesses, citizens, community groups, foundations and the mass media. Such governance for health is dispersed and horizontal. It promotes joint action for a common interest by health and non-health sectors.

Governments at all levels are considering establishing formal structures and processes that support coherence and intersectoral problem-solving and address power imbalances between sectors. Structures and mechanisms that enable collaboration need to support synergistic policies for health and well-being. In this sense, effective multilevel governance is just as important as intersectoral and participatory governance. Governance and policy processes for health need to be transparent and open, ensuring as broad participation as possible by various sectors, levels and interest groups. Adaptive policies need to be sufficiently resilient to respond to complexity and to be prepared for uncertainty.

Creating the awareness and capacity to make health objectives part of society's overall socioeconomic and human development is an essential task. All policy fields, not only health, need to reform their ways of working and employ new forms and approaches to policy-making and implementation at the global, regional and local levels. Importantly, health is not the only field that requires action in other sectors: there are bilateral and multilateral needs for synergistically developing and implementing jointly owned policy across all sectors.

Achieving intersectoral action within the machinery of government is clearly challenging. The reasons include the complexity of the issues involved, the wicked nature of the challenges and the inherent inflexibility of bureaucratic organizational systems. The distribution of influence and resources within society, conflicts of interest within government, a lack of incentives and lack of commitment at the highest level also drive the challenges.

This new concept of governance for health brings together and extends the prior notions of intersectoral action and healthy public policy within the more comprehensive and linked notions of whole-of-society and whole-of-government responsibility for health. Intrinsic here is a health-in-all-policies approach that advocates putting health higher up the policy agenda, strengthening the policy dialogue on health and its determinants, and building accountability for health outcomes. Health impact assessment and economic evaluation are valuable tools in assessing the potential effects of policies and can also be used to assess the effects on quality. These approaches emphasize not only the need for better coordination and integration among government activities on health but also reaching out beyond government to others, thereby achieving a joint contribution to overarching societal goals such as prosperity, well-being, equity and sustainability.

Health governance

Health 2020 refers to governance of the health sector itself as health governance. This involves being responsible for developing and implementing national and subnational health strategies; setting health goals and targets for improving health; delivering high-quality and effective health care services; and ensuring core public health functions. It also means being responsible for considering how policy decisions affect other sectors and stakeholders.

Health governance generates incentives to promote better performance, accountability and transparency, as well as full user involvement, through an institutional structure that enables resources, providers and their services to be organized and managed towards accomplishing a common policy and national health goals. Also required is a common understanding of the (evidence-informed) means to attain these objectives.

Health ministries are increasingly engaged in initiating intersectoral approaches for health and acting as health brokers and advocates. As emphasized in the Tallinn Charter *(24)*, the health sector must engage in working with other sectors in ways that are mutually supportive and constructive, in engagements that are "win-win" for overall societal public health goals, in addition to delivering individual health care services. The health sector also has a partnership role towards other sectors when strengthening health can contribute to achieving their goals. At the United Nations High-level Meeting on the Prevention and Control of Noncommunicable Diseases and in the World Health Assembly, all countries have endorsed such collaborative approaches – referred to as whole-of-government and whole-of-society approaches.

Smart governance

Although any normative approach to governance may be contested, the principles and processes of good governance have been considered in relation to countries, for example through the World Bank's Worldwide governance indicators project *(52)*, which shows important correlations between good governance and health. Both governance for health and health governance are based around a system of values and principles referred to as good governance. Smart governance describes the mechanisms chosen to reach results based on the principles of good governance.

Research indicates the need for a combination of governance approaches – hierarchical, dispersed and participatory – to benefit health and well-being. Five types of smart governance for health may be considered.

- *Governing through collaboration*. Consideration needs to be given to the processes of collaboration, the virtuous circle between communication, trust, commitment and understanding, the choice of tools and mechanisms available and the need for transparency and accountability.
- *Governing through citizen engagement*. As governance becomes more diffused throughout society, working directly with the public can strengthen transparency and accountability. Partnering and empowering the public are also crucial in ensuring that values are upheld. Technology, particularly networked social media, is a driving force enabling citizens to change how governments and health systems do business. Within these complex relationships, participation, transparency and accountability become engines for innovation.
- *Governing through a mixture of regulation and persuasion*. Governing is becoming more fluid, multilevel, multistakeholder and adaptive. Traditional

hierarchical means of governance are increasingly being complemented by other mechanisms, such as soft power and soft law. These include self-regulation, governance by persuasion, alliances, networks and open methods of coordination. Health promotion approaches are being revisited with the growing influence of nudge policies *(53)*. Hierarchical multilevel regulations that extend from global to local levels, such as the WHO Framework Convention on Tobacco Control, are becoming more common, affecting many dimensions of individuals' lifestyles, behaviour and everyday lives.

- *Governing through independent agencies and expert bodies*. Such entities play an increasingly important role in providing evidence, observing ethical boundaries, expanding accountability and strengthening democratic accountability in health, related to such fields as privacy, risk assessment, quality control, health technology assessment and health impact assessment.
- *Governing through adaptive policies, resilient structures and foresight*. Whole-of-government approaches need to be adaptive and mirror the complexities of causality, because complex and wicked problems have no simple linear causality or solution. Decentralized decision-making and self-organizing or social networking help stakeholders respond quickly to unanticipated events in innovative ways. Interventions should be iterative and integrate continuous learning, multistakeholder knowledge-gathering and sharing, and mechanisms to encourage further deliberation or automatic policy adjustment. Policy interventions in one area can have unintended consequences in another, and studies indicate the value of promoting a wide variation of smaller-scale interventions at the local and community levels for the same problem, to encourage learning and adaptation. Anticipatory governance with participatory foresight mechanisms can also support societal resilience by shifting policy from risks to addressing more fundamental systemic challenges and jointly deliberating the social and value- and science-based dimensions of public policy.

Working together on common priorities for health

The Health 2020 policy framework proposes four common areas for policy action based on the categories for priority-setting and programmes in WHO agreed by Member States at the global level and aligned to address the special requirements and experiences of the European Region. These also build on relevant WHO strategies and action plans at the regional and global levels:

- investing in health through a life-course approach and empowering people;
- tackling Europe's major disease burdens of noncommunicable and communicable diseases;
- strengthening people-centred health systems, public health capacity, and emergency preparedness surveillance and response; and
- creating resilient communities and supportive environments.

The four priority areas are not discrete areas of action but are frequently interdependent and mutually supportive. For example, taking action on the life-course and empowering people will help to contain the epidemic of noncommunicable diseases, as will strengthening public health capacity. Governments achieve greater health effects when they link up policies, investment and services and focus on reducing inequality. The WHO Regional Office for Europe will step up its role as a resource for developing policy based on examples of and evidence about such integrated approaches.

Addressing these priorities requires combining governance approaches – hierarchical, dispersed and participatory – to make health and well-being possible for everyone. Such governance will anticipate change, foster innovation, and be oriented towards investing in promoting health and preventing disease. New approaches to governance for health will include governing through collaboration, through citizen engagement, through a mix of regulation and persuasion, and through independent agencies and expert bodies. The latter, in particular, reflect the increasing function of assessing evidence, overseeing ethical boundaries, expanding transparency and strengthening democratic accountability in such fields as privacy, risk assessment and health impact assessment.

The Health 2020 policy framework also recognizes that many health policy decisions have to be taken under conditions of uncertain and imperfect knowledge. What works best in tackling such complex problems as obesity, multiple morbidities and neurodegenerative diseases is not yet clear. Context is also important, since what may work in one health system or country may not be exportable without appropriate adaptation. The system effects of many aspects of health system reform also cannot be fully predicted. Studies note the value of promoting a wide range of smaller-scale yet multifaceted interventions focused on problem-solving at the local and community levels, to encourage learning and adaptation.

Investing in health through a life-course approach and empowering people

Supporting good health and its social determinants throughout the lifespan leads to increasing healthy life expectancy and a longevity dividend, both of which can yield important economic, societal and individual benefits. The demographic transformation requires an effective life-course strategy that gives priority to new approaches to empowering people and building resilience and capacity, so as to promote health and prevent disease. Children with a good start in life learn better and have more productive lives; adults with control over their lives have greater capacity for economic and social participation and living healthier lives; and healthy older people can continue to contribute actively to society. Healthy and active ageing, which starts at birth, is a policy priority and a major research priority.

Health promotion programmes based on principles of engagement and empowerment offer real benefits for health and its determinants. These can include creating better conditions for living, improving life skills and health literacy, supporting independent living and making the healthier choice the easier choice. This means making pregnancies safe; giving people a good start in life; promoting safety and well-being and giving protection during childhood and for young people; promoting good quality and healthy workplaces; and supporting active and healthy ageing. Providing healthy food and a safe and sustainable environment throughout the lifespan is a priority, given the growing epidemic in noncommunicable diseases and their determinants. Investing in healthy settings initiatives offers unique opportunities to reinforce health literacy.

Healthy women, mothers and babies

Situation analysis

Women's reproductive years have enormous effects on their general health and well-being, and the lives of a mother and her baby are inextricably linked. Safe family planning, safe pregnancy and childbirth, and breastfeeding are prerequisites for growing up healthily, but for many women, pregnancy and childbirth are still a time of risk. Although the maternal mortality ratio was almost halved in the European Region as a whole from 1990 to 2006, progress has been uneven, and striking inequalities persist between and within countries in the European Region. Maternity can lead to complications: for every woman who dies in childbirth globally, at least 20 others are estimated to experience injury, infection and disability *(54)*.

Women need to be empowered to control reproduction. Some women cannot choose pregnancy and motherhood, but the alternatives pose difficulties of their own. Many countries have great unmet need for safe and effective contraception, and the European Region has the highest levels of induced abortion of any WHO region, with unsafe abortion causing up to 30% of maternal deaths in some countries *(55,56)*.

The major direct causes of maternal morbidity and mortality include haemorrhage, infection, high blood pressure, unsafe abortion and obstructed labour. These can be prevented and treated with basic, cost-effective interventions, but not all women in the WHO European Region have access to the care or services they need.

The age of sexual debut is decreasing in many countries in the European Region. In many cases, unsafe sex leads to sexually transmitted infections and unintended pregnancies. Women and men are planning and having children at later ages; this increases the risk of congenital malformation, infertility, medically assisted reproduction, high-risk pregnancies because of chronic diseases, and other health problems *(57,58)*.

There are substantial inequities in the Region within and between countries in access to skilled workers at delivery, during antenatal care, and in family planning and other reproductive health services. A mother's educational level, her health and nutrition, her socioeconomic status, the prevalent gender norms and roles, and the quality of health and social services she receives profoundly affect her chances of a successful pregnancy and outcome *(59)*.

The infant mortality rate for the European Region has also fallen by more than 50% since 1990, but again countries differ substantially, with a 25-fold difference between the countries with highest and lowest rates. For example, the infant mortality rate in the central Asian republics and Kazakhstan is more than twice the rate for the European Region and more than four times the rate for the 15 countries that were EU members before 2004 (EU15). Children have the highest risk of dying during the first 28 days of life, and 75% of neonatal deaths occur during the first week of life *(60,61)*.

The main causes of death among newborn babies are prematurity and low birth weight, infections, asphyxia, birth trauma and congenital abnormalities; these account for nearly 80% of deaths in this age group. They are intrinsically socioeconomic in origin – linked to the health and social conditions of the mother and the care received before, during and immediately after birth. In general, the proportions of deaths attributed to prematurity and congenital disorders increase as the neonatal mortality rate decreases, and the proportions caused by infections and asphyxia decline as care improves *(62)*.

Solutions that work

Contextual factors such as a healthy environment, women's empowerment, education and poverty play an important role in reducing maternal, newborn and child mortality levels, as does care provided through health systems. Although both care and contextual interventions contribute to reducing maternal mortality, this may depend more on the efforts of health systems and less on contextual factors than does child mortality. When the context is particularly challenging, even strong health systems can have only limited effects on mortality; conversely, when there is an enabling context for health, a poor health system could substantially hold back mortality reduction.

Access to sexuality education, family planning services and safe abortion reduces the number of unintended pregnancies and mortality and morbidity from abortion without influencing the fertility rate.

Introducing the WHO Effective Perinatal Care training package *(63)* has reduced maternal and perinatal mortality and reduced inequalities. Together with the introduction of maternal and perinatal audit, the package has been demonstrated to lead to better, healthier childbirth. The development and implementation of national clinical guidelines and a perinatal referral system have resulted in a decrease in maternal and perinatal mortality. In addition, better registration of perinatal deaths has provided a basis for strategic planning.

Providing well-known and effective health interventions during pregnancy, at birth and during the first week of life could prevent two thirds of newborn deaths, reduce maternal mortality and provide a better start for those babies that survive. The interventions and approaches that can help save the lives of mothers and babies work even where resources are scarce. Evidence is mounting to show that investing in early childhood development is one of the most powerful measures countries can take in reducing the escalating burden of chronic disease *(26,64–73)*.

Breastfeeding is an important aspect of caring for infants and young children. It leads to improved nutrition and physical growth, reduced susceptibility to common childhood illnesses and better resistance to cope with them, a reduced risk of certain noncommunicable diseases in later life, stimulating bonding with the caregiver and psychosocial development.

Relevant WHO strategies at the global and regional levels are those relating to sexual and reproductive health *(74,75)*, the prevention and control of sexually transmitted infections *(76)* and infant and young child feeding *(77)*. WHO's work is linked with that of achieving the United Nations Millennium Development Goals *(69,78)*, particularly those to reduce child mortality and improve maternal health. Millennium Development Goal 1 on eradicating extreme poverty and hunger includes a focus on infant and young child feeding, and Millennium Development Goal 3 promotes gender equality and the empowerment of women. The Global Strategy for Women's and Children's Health was launched at the United Nations in 2010 and recognized that the health of women and children is key to progress on all development goals *(79–81)*. To improve global reporting, oversight and accountability for women's and children's health, WHO convened the Commission on Information and Accountability for Women's and Children's Health in 2010.

Healthy children and healthy adolescents

Situation analysis

The European Region includes the countries with some of the lowest child mortality rates in the world, and most children and adolescents in the WHO European Region enjoy a high standard of health and well-being. However, it also includes some wide variation: the rates in countries with the highest mortality among children younger than five years are 20–30 times the rates of the lowest.

The mortality rate in the European Region among children younger than five years is 9.81 per 1000 live births. Mortality among children younger than 15 years has decreased for all groups of countries in the European Region, and mortality among children younger than five years is now the lowest of any WHO region, although it can differ substantially between countries. For example, child mortality rates are declining more slowly in the countries in the Commonwealth of Independent States (CIS),[5] where a child born is three times as likely to die before the age of five years as a child born in an EU country.

The leading causes of death of children younger than five years in the European Region are neonatal conditions, pneumonia and diarrhoea. Almost half the deaths are associated with undernutrition. Children are also at risk from hazardous environments, obesity and unhealthy lifestyles. Poor environments aggravate socioeconomic disparities in cities. Marked differences in mortality rates among children younger than five years between urban and rural areas and between households with the lowest and highest incomes have been demonstrated where data exist *(27,69,82–85)*.

Suicide and accidents result in considerable deaths and disability among young people. Every day, more than 300 young people in the European Region die from largely preventable causes. Almost 10% of 18-year-olds in the European Region have depression. Injuries are the leading cause of death among young people; road traffic injuries are the leading cause of death and the leading cause of injury among people aged 10–24 years *(86–90)*. Young men are more affected by suicide and accidents in all countries and across all socioeconomic groups *(91)*.

A good start in life establishes the basis for healthy life. A good start is characterized by the following: a mother was in a position to make reproductive health choices, is healthy during pregnancy, gives birth to a baby of healthy weight, the baby experiences warm and responsive relationships in infancy, has access to high-quality child care and early education, and lives in a stimulating environment that allow safe access to outdoor play. Evidence shows that high-quality early child services, with effects on parenting, can compensate for the effects on early child development of social disadvantage.

The first year of life is crucial for healthy physical and mental development. Children and adolescents need safe and supportive environments: clean air, safe housing, nutritious food, clean water and a healthy way of life. They also need access to friendly and age-appropriate services. Promoting physical, cognitive, social and emotional development is crucial for all children, from the earliest years. Children who experience a good start are likely to do well at school, attain better paid employment, and enjoy better physical and mental health in adulthood.

The foundational strengths for well-being, such as problem-solving, emotional regulation and physical safety, are the positive underpinnings of early child

[5] The CIS consisted of Armenia, Azerbaijan, Belarus, Georgia, Kazakhstan, Kyrgyzstan, the Republic of Moldova, the Russian Federation, Tajikistan, Turkmenistan, Ukraine and Uzbekistan when the data were collected.

health and development. Developing these skills and optimizing well-being in early childhood establish the basis for ongoing well-being across the life-course.

Children born into disadvantaged home and family circumstances have a higher risk of poor growth and development. Optimizing health and well-being in later life requires investing in positive early childhood experiences and development. Good social, emotional and mental health helps to protect children against emotional and behavioural problems, violence and crime, teenage pregnancy and misusing drugs and alcohol, and determines how well they do in school *(92–100)*.

Many serious diseases and types of exposure to risk factors (such as tobacco use and poor eating and exercise habits) in adulthood originate in childhood and adolescence. For example, tobacco use, mental ill health, sexually transmitted infections including HIV, and poor eating and exercise habits may all lead to illness or premature death later in life. The prevalence of overweight among children younger than 16 years is between 10% and 20% in the European Region, with rates higher among children in southern Europe. The dietary habits of young people are not optimal for health: they include fruit and vegetable consumption below recommended levels and high consumption of sweetened beverages. Physical activity levels decrease during adolescence, more markedly among girls. Smoking prevalence at age 13 years is 5%, rising to 19% by age 15 years in the European Region. Almost two thirds of 16-year-olds have consumed alcohol in the previous 30 days. The percentage of 15-year-olds reporting that they have experienced sexual intercourse ranges from 12% to 38% across countries in the European Region *(58,101–103)*. The use of condoms and other contraceptives differs between countries, as well as between boys and girls.

Adolescence is usually a time of good health for both girls and boys, with opportunities for growth and development. Today young people mature physically and grow up at an earlier age than hitherto. Nevertheless, adolescence can also be time of risk, particularly with regard to unsafe sexual activity, substance use and accidents. The social and economic environment in which adolescents grow up often determines the behaviour they develop during adolescence *(93)*. Research shows that boys and girls differ in their exposure and vulnerability to health risks and conditions such as depressive disorders, injuries, substance abuse, eating disorders, sexually transmitted infections, violence, suicide and self-inflicted injuries *(91)*.

Solutions that work

Much of the morbidity and mortality among children and adolescents is preventable. Low-cost, effective measures could prevent two thirds of deaths. Several childhood illnesses can be prevented by immunization and relatively simple, low-cost measures. The WHO Integrated Management of Childhood Illnesses (IMCI) strategy promotes a package of simple, affordable and effective interventions for combined management of the major childhood illnesses and malnutrition, including antibiotics, treatment of anaemia, immunization and promoting breastfeeding *(104,105)*.

Measures to control tobacco use and the harmful use of alcohol need to emphasize protecting children through effective population-level measures and regulatory frameworks such as banning advertising, banning sales to minors, promoting smoke-free environments and pricing policies. Children are vulnerable and exposed to marketing pressure, and interventions can reduce the effects on children of the marketing of foods high in saturated fat, *trans*-fatty acids, free sugar or salt. Environmental measures can be put in place to promote physical activity: for example, through urban design and planning the school day.

A strategic focus on healthy living for younger people is particularly valuable. Numerous factors influence children's social and emotional well-being, from their individual make-up and family background to the community within which they live and society at large. As a result, a broader multiagency strategy is required, to which people themselves can contribute. A broad range of stakeholders can be mobilized to support programmes that promote health, including generational activities. For young people, these can include policies to improve the social and economic status of children living in disadvantaged circumstances *(91,92,95,106–109)*; whole-school approaches to school-based activities to develop and protect children's social and emotional well-being, including school-based health literacy programmes; peer-to-peer education; and the development of youth organizations. Integrating work on mental and sexual health into these programmes and activities is particularly important.

Relevant WHO strategies at the global and regional levels are those relating to child and adolescent health and development *(110)*, preventing and controlling sexually transmitted infections *(76)*, infant and young child feeding *(77)* and the Children's Environment and Health Action Plan for Europe *(83)*. Work is under way to achieve relevant the United Nations Millennium Development Goals, such as Goal 1 to reduce child mortality and Goal 2 to achieve universal primary education. Strong evidence indicates the need for gender-responsive actions to improve adolescent health in several areas such as mental health, obesity, injuries, HIV, chronic diseases, sexual and reproductive health, violence and well-being *(91)*.

Healthy adults

Situation analysis

The adult stage of life entails such events as taking up employment, parenting, citizenship and caring for parents. For many adults, there is challenge in achieving work–life balance and in reconciling private and professional responsibilities, with women and single parents struggling the most. Women face disadvantage regarding access to and participation in the labour market, and men face disadvantage regarding participation in family life.

Predetermined social models tend to presuppose that men are mainly responsible for paid work derived from economic activity and that women are mainly responsible for unpaid work related to looking after a family. In many countries and some cultures in the European Region, traditional gender norms still prevent women from taking up gainful employment and earning income. There is still a huge imbalance between men and women in the distribution of family and domestic responsibilities. Parenthood negatively affects employment for women: many women opt for flexible working arrangements or give up work altogether, affecting women's career development, the wage gap between men and women and pension rights.

Parenting policies and services should empower women with children to take control over their lives, support the health and development of their children and support a greater parenting role for men. In particular, family-friendly employment policies should be strengthened by introducing more flexible working hours – without turning to insecure short-term contracts – and making affordable child care available, to help parents combine work with their parental responsibilities.

The ability to successfully reconcile private and work life, to achieve an optimal work–life balance, has implications for fertility rates and demographic renewal.

With an ageing population, women and men frequently have a double burden of caring for children and caring for older dependants. Couples and individuals need to be able to decide freely and responsibly the number, spacing and timing of their children and to have the information and means to do so. Sexual health and the reproductive years tremendously affect women's and men's general health and well-being, but in some parts of the Region, sexual and reproductive health needs may still be considered too private or culturally sensitive to be addressed properly.

Sexual health care aims to enhance life and personal relationships and not merely to provide counselling and care on reproduction and sexually transmitted infections. Relevant WHO strategies include those promoting sexual health and reproductive choice *(74,75)*.

Numerous social changes in the European Region affect adults disproportionately at different stages of life. A good-quality job with a high level of job control and a correct balance between effort and reward is an important prerequisite for health. For many young people, unemployment is still high and instability in early employment has become the norm, often with adverse effects on fertility and forming families. For older workers, standard retirement trajectories have eroded and become replaced by instability of employment late in people's careers and various pathways into early retirement. Women's increasing integration into paid employment is often associated with atypical forms of work.

Lack of control over work and home life can harm health. Accumulation of psychosocial risk can increase long-term stress and the chances of premature death. Both jobs with high demands on employees and jobs with low employee control carry risk. Health suffers when people have little control over their work, little opportunity to use their skills and low authority to make decisions.

Unemployment, insecurity, discrimination and exclusion from work increase the risk of physical and mental disorders. Long-term unemployment is a grave concern for long-term health outcomes.

Solutions that work

Promoting the well-being of adults in the European Region requires a variety of approaches. Social innovation approaches that involve communities in policy-making processes can be used to optimize well-being by engaging citizens in addressing an array of social and well-being issues and proposing solutions that are desirable to use and enrich people's daily lives. Workplace health promotion that is designed not just to prevent disease but also to optimize employee well-being can benefit employees and employers. Improved conditions of work, with mechanisms that enable people to influence the design and improvement of their work, lead to a healthier, more productive workplace.

Governments should make every effort to avoid unemployment (particularly long-term unemployment), insecurity, discrimination and exclusion from work. Key health-related measures include active labour market programmes, promoting the use of permanent contracts for employment, adapting the physical and psychosocial working environment to meet the needs of individual employees, increasing the influence that employees have over their work individually and collectively, and strengthening occupational health services. As retirement ages are likely to rise, the needs of an ageing workforce must also be taken into account.

Social protection policies in the form of active labour market policies and return-to-work interventions can have a protective health effect in times of economic downturn and rising unemployment *(111)*. EU mortality trends during recessions in the past three decades indicate that countries can avoid a rise in suicide rates by spending US$ 200 per person per year on more active labour market programmes designed to improve peoples' chances of gaining employment and protecting those in employment.

In low- and medium-income countries, policy actions will include promoting sustainable green economic growth; transferring knowledge and skills; increasing employability, especially among young people; achieving greater job stability among the most vulnerable people; reducing exposure to unhealthy work and the associated risks of disease and injury; and managing health risks by enforcing national regulations and providing good occupational health services.

In high-income countries, policy actions will include maintaining high levels of employment through green, sustainable economies; preserving standards of decent work and social protection policies; developing standardized tools for monitoring and risk management; and implementing known methods to improve safe and healthy work, with priority given to high-risk groups, including unemployed people.

In achieving work–life balance, a number of supportive measures can be put in place including granting family-related leave; improving the provision of child care; organizing working time to include flexible arrangements; abolishing conditions that lead to wage differences between men and women; harmonizing school and working hours; and reviewing the opening hours of shops. Employment policies should also provide measures that encourage more equitable sharing between men and women of leave for child care and care of older people. Differences between countries demonstrate what can be achieved in supportive social policy.

The EU's Lisbon Strategy *(112)* recognized the importance of furthering all aspects of equal opportunities. Improved reconciliation of family and working life is a guideline of the European Employment Strategy and is included in the European process for combating poverty and promoting social inclusion. WHO resolutions relating to social inclusion, gender equality, and poverty and health at the global and regional levels are also relevant *(113)*.

Healthy older people

Situation analysis

Overall, longer life expectancy for both women and men is a major achievement, where health and social policies have played an important role. As life expectancy increases, more people are living past 65 years of age and into very old age, thus dramatically increasing the numbers of older people. By 2050, more than one quarter (27%) of the population is expected to be 65 years and older. There are 2.5 women for each man among those aged 85 years or over, and this imbalance is projected to increase by 2050 *(70)*.

Although women in the European Region live on average 7.5 years longer than men, they live a greater share of their lives in poor health than men. Since women also have higher disability rates, women comprise the vast majority of very old people who need ongoing health care and social support *(114)*.

As individuals age, noncommunicable diseases become the leading causes of morbidity, disability and mortality, and multiple morbidities become more common. Socioeconomic status greatly affects health with, for example, morbidity often higher in later life among people with lower-status occupations. A great proportion of overall health care needs and costs are concentrated in the last few years of life.

If people are empowered to remain healthy into old age, severe morbidity can often be compressed into a few short months before death. Nevertheless, any possible compression of morbidity would be too small to offset the effect of rising numbers of older people, so the number of older people with disabilities will also rise. About 20% of people aged 70 years or older and 50% of people aged 85 years and older report difficulties in performing activities of daily living such as bathing, dressing and toileting, as well as other activities such as housekeeping, laundry and taking medication. Restriction of mobility is common, as is sensory impairment. About one third of people 75–84 years old report difficulties in hearing during conversation with other people, and about one fifth have problems reading daily newspapers or books.

Currently, many countries in the European Region have, in global terms, extremely low fertility rates and very high life expectancy *(70)*. Consequently, the support and care of an increasing number of older people depends on an ever-reducing number of people of working age. Care of older people is still considered a familial obligation rather than a government responsibility, in many countries, and most informal caregivers are women. The state of development and extent of the care of older people differs more widely between countries in the European Region than for other health and social policy programmes. Formal social care for older people is more likely to be available in urban areas, while access to and the quality of nursing homes differs widely in Europe. Privacy and high-quality care may be limited, access to mainstream health care may be limited, medication may be inappropriate and preventive measures may fail.

Although increased longevity is a triumph, it can also present a challenge. Projections foresee an increase in overall age-related public spending (pensions, health and long-term care) of about 4–5% of gross domestic product (GDP) between 2004 and 2050 for the EU15, for example *(115)*. The economic impact of ageing populations on public-sector spending during the coming decades can be substantially mitigated if longer lifetimes are accompanied by parallel increases in the age of retirement.

Health and activity in older age are the sum of the living circumstances and actions of an individual during his or her whole lifespan. Experiences throughout the life-course affect well-being in older age – lifelong financial hardship is associated with worse health outcomes later in life, and people who have been married all their adult lives outlive those who have not.

Older people are not a homogeneous group: individual diversity increases with age, and the rate of functional decline is determined not only by factors related to individual behaviour but also by social, economic or environmental factors that individuals may not be able to modify. For example, age discrimination in access to high-quality services is widespread, and inequities in the living conditions and well-being of older people are greater than among younger people because of substantial differences in the family situation of individual older people and systematic inequities in pension incomes and accumulated assets *(116)*.

Early age at retirement, experiencing a job loss and experiencing traumatic life events, especially later in life, are associated with poorer well-being in middle and later life. Social support, especially social relationships with family and friends, is one of the most important factors influencing the quality of life among older people. Gender (women), single marital status, lack of material resources (such as access to a car) and poor health are all associated with less social contact in older adults.

The key needs of older people include being autonomous, having a voice and belonging to the community. One of the most powerful strategies for promoting health and well-being in old age is preventing loneliness and isolation, in which support from families and peers plays a key role. Initiatives for active and healthy ageing can benefit health and the quality of life. To support public authorities in implementing healthy ageing policies under the Health 2020 framework, Member States in the European Region have endorsed a complementary *Strategy and action plan for healthy ageing in Europe, 2012–2020 (117)*.

The decline in functional capacity among older people is potentially reversible and can be influenced at any age through individual and public policy measures, such as promoting age-friendly living environments.

The life-course approach to healthy ageing gives people a good start in life and influences how they age, by giving them the capability to live a better life and empowering them to adopt healthier lifestyles throughout their lives and adapt to age-associated changes. Older people need to be empowered and encouraged to have healthy lifestyles. This can be facilitated by providing opportunities for exercise, healthy nutrition and smoking cessation, for example. Effective measures to promote healthy ageing include legislation, social and economic policies that provide for adequate social protection – including income support and supplementation, policies for supportive transport, neighbourhood and urban planning and public health promotion work on risk factors.

Putting an appropriate mix of services in place (such as health and social services, technical aids and support for informal care) is key to making health and long-term care systems sustainable in the future *(118)*. Creating environments and services that enable people to stay healthy longer and stay active in the labour market will be crucial to reducing or containing long-term unemployment, disability benefits and early retirement. Adapting building design, urban planning and transport systems to meet the needs of older people and people with disabilities can maintain independent living, reduce the impact of disability and support social networks.

The promotion of the health and well-being of older people may be mainstreamed into policies and initiatives on active, dignified and healthy ageing, on reducing health inequities, on retirement and on promoting the rights of people with disabilities. Key actions include ensuring that older people are involved in developing health policy and in making decisions about their own treatment and care; developing tools to promote health literacy and disease self-management, including among family caregivers; reducing mental health risks among older people with chronic physical disorders; addressing negative societal stereotypes about old age through mass media work; and implementing independent quality control measures to monitor the quality of the services provided in institutions.

Vaccination is effective in both children and older people in reducing the morbidity and mortality resulting from several infectious diseases. Among older people, screening for treatable diseases such as breast cancer can reduce premature morbidity and mortality.

Palliative care affirms life and regards dying as a normal process and intends neither to hasten nor to prolong death. It provides relief from pain and other distressing symptoms and should be offered as needs develop and before they become unmanageable *(119)*. Traditionally, high-quality care at the end of life has mainly been provided for people with cancer in inpatient hospices, but this kind of care now needs to be provided for people with a wider range of diseases, including the increasing number of people with dementia, and needs to reach into people's homes and into nursing and residential homes within the community (120). Palliative care offers a support system to help people live as actively as possible until death and to help the family members cope during the person's illness and in their own bereavement.

A World Health Assembly resolution on active ageing *(121)* called on Member States to ensure the highest attainable standard of health and well-being for their older citizens, and a recent WHO Executive Board resolution *(122)* included a focus on developing age-friendly primary health care. The Second World Assembly on Ageing was held in Madrid, Spain in 2002 and led to the adoption of the International Plan of Action on Ageing *(123)*. WHO developed *Active ageing: a policy framework (124)* as a contribution to the Assembly.

Public spending at the boundary between health and social care has important efficiency gains that are largely not being realized, with evidence accumulating about cost-effective interventions to avoid emergency hospital admissions and long lengths of stay or how telemedicine and telecare can best be harnessed. Health care and long-term care need to be integrated better, and aspects related to dignity and human rights in long-term care need to be improved. The quality of services also needs to be improved through quality assessment and assurance mechanisms and through new models of care coordination and integration, including care pathways that provide tailored packages of health and social care.

Better policies to combat noncommunicable diseases over the life-course are key to healthy ageing, as are age-friendly communities and better access to high-quality health and social services for older people. Supporting more people so they can remain active at work for longer and redistributing work over the life-course can both contribute to healthy ageing and make health and welfare policies sustainable in the long term. The increasing number of examples with regard to good practice coordination and integration of care, including bridging the gap between health and social services, can help countries in reforming health care with the aim of considerably improving the coverage and social protection of older people with care needs.

Vulnerability, vulnerable groups and health

Situation analysis

Vulnerability sometimes refers simply to a lack of physical and/or mental resilience among individual people, but here the context is broader – vulnerability to both social adversity and ill health. This results from exclusionary processes that operate differentially across the whole of society and give rise to the social gradient in health. Although social exclusion is a dynamic and gradual phenomenon and actions should focus on addressing exclusionary processes, identifying individuals or groups who are socially excluded and considering them in both research and policy-making are equally important. Two specific groups are highlighted, migrants and Roma, to illustrate many of the issues faced by vulnerable groups in general

Migrants Migration in Europe today involves a diverse group of people, including regular and irregular migrants, victims of human trafficking, asylum-seekers, refugees, displaced people and returnees. Many migrate for economic reasons. Overall, 75 million migrants live in the WHO European Region, amounting to 8% of the total population and 39% of all migrants worldwide *(78)*. Most migrants in the European Region are young adults. Women comprise half of all migrants and are often overrepresented in vulnerable groups, such as victims of human trafficking for sexual exploitation *(125)*.

There are substantial variations between groups, countries and health conditions. Nevertheless, the burden of ill health among excluded migrant groups is often unacceptably large *(126)*. Where figures exist, they generally indicate lower life expectancy for migrants, and some communities also show increased rates of infant mortality. Migrants' illnesses are largely similar to those of the rest of the population, although some groups may have a higher prevalence of health problems, including communicable diseases; poor nutrition; high rates of alcohol and drug abuse; reproductive and sexual ill health; occupational health problems; and mental disorders *(127–129)*.

The vulnerability of most migrants leaves them exposed to hazardous working environments, poor housing, labour exploitation and inadequate access to health care. Occupational accident rates are about twice as high for migrant workers as for native workers in the European Region *(126)*.

The health conditions and environment at the migrants' place of origin, such as a high prevalence of tuberculosis or HIV infection, determine many baseline health characteristics, with health risks increasing during the migratory journey, for example owing to traumatic experiences *(130)*. After arrival, poverty and social exclusion exert the greatest influence on health outcomes, with the availability, accessibility, acceptability and quality of services in the host environment influencing the health of migrants *(126)*. On arrival, a variety of factors may increase psychosocial vulnerability and hinder successful integration. Migrants may experience obstacles in accessing services because of stigmatization, lack of information about services and lack of information in other than the predominant languages of host countries.

Roma

About 12–15 million Roma live in the European Region, and an estimated 10 million live in the EU alone. Roma are estimated to account for 10% of the population of Bulgaria, 9% in Slovakia and 8% in Romania, and these proportions are likely to increase *(126,131)*.

There are indications that life expectancy among Roma communities is 10–15 years lower than average, the rates of infant mortality are increased and the levels of maternal and child mortality and morbidity are alarmingly high *(131–133)*.

Higher rates of illness have been reported among Roma populations than among majority populations, with higher rates of type 2 diabetes, coronary artery disease and obesity among adults and of nutritional deficiencies and malnutrition among children. For example, many Roma women in settlements in Serbia are undernourished (51%) and smoke tobacco (almost all), and a United Nations Development Programme survey of vulnerability found that 50% of Roma children face malnutrition risks more than twice monthly, in contrast to 6% of majority children *(134–136)*.

A disproportionate number of Roma have low income in many countries, and evidence suggests that this leads to a concentration of Roma among the people with the lowest incomes. Exclusion linked to discrimination against Roma may be an independent risk factor for poverty *(132,137)*.

Evidence indicates significant inequity in health system access and health status between Roma and majority populations. For instance, data on antenatal care coverage, low birth weight, prevalence of breastfeeding, maternal smoking, nutritional status and vaccination rates reveal marked inequities between the Roma and the majority population, including (in some contexts) when Roma are compared with the poorest quintile of the general population *(138,139)*.

Solutions that work

Since the health problems of migrants and others who are vulnerable can result from or be worsened by their disadvantageous social position, measures that combat socially exclusionary processes are likely to have the most fundamental effect on their health. Furthermore, policies should address inequities in the state of health of migrants, Roma and others made vulnerable through exclusionary processes, and in the accessibility and quality of health and social services available to them. Many of the strategies for achieving this are not specific to such groups as the Roma, but are similar to those needed for ethnic minorities and others subject to multiple exclusionary processes in general. They include training health care workers in working with minority and marginalized populations, involving those populations in designing, implementing and evaluating health programmes, and improving health information systems so that data are collected and presented in an ethnically disaggregated format. Integrated policy approaches designed to tackle the multiple causes of social exclusion are the most successful *(140)*.

Many of the health and socioeconomic challenges associated with migration are the product of global inequity, and action that focuses solely on host countries will be less effective than integrated global programmes designed to mitigate the factors in the country and region both of origin and of destination.

Migrants also frequently confront gender-specific challenges, particularly in the context of maternal, newborn and child health, sexual and reproductive health, and violence. Migrants should have early access to reproductive health services, preventive health services and health promotion, screening and diagnostic care, as well as prenatal and obstetric services. Special attention should be paid to women and girls who have been trafficked, as many have been exposed to gender-based violence.

WHO resolutions adopted at global and regional levels relating to social inclusion and poverty and health are relevant to vulnerable people. These include the World Health Assembly resolution on reducing health inequities through action on the social determinants of health *(47)* and work following up Regional Committee resolution EUR/RC52/R7 on poverty and health *(141)*, such as that addressing health inequities linked to migration and ethnicity *(126)*.

Specifically on the health of migrants, a World Health Assembly resolution in 2008 *(142)* was followed up by a WHO/International Organization for Migration global consultation on an operational framework during the Spanish EU Presidency in 2010 *(143)*. The need for coordinated and sustained international action is being picked up through various policy processes and conferences, with outcome documents, such as the Bratislava Declaration on Health, Human Rights and Migration signed by Council of Europe Member countries in 2007 *(144)* and recommendations on mobility, migration and access to health care adopted by the Council of Europe Committee of Ministers in 2011 *(145)*. The International Convention on the Protection of the Rights of All Migrant Workers and Members of their Families *(146)* provides a broader framework for the universal human right to health without discrimination.

The Decade of Roma Inclusion 2005–2015 is a political commitment by European governments to improve the socioeconomic status and social inclusion of Roma, and health is a priority area of focus together with education, employment and housing. In 2011, the European Commission launched an EU Framework for National Roma Integration Strategies by 2020, which requests that all EU countries develop and implement targeted strategies for promoting integration in health, housing, education and employment *(131)*. Other relevant work includes the European Council communication on solidarity in health and the European Council's conclusions on Roma *(147)*.

Gender equity through the life-course

Situation analysis

A gender approach is needed to understand and tackle socioeconomic and health inequities. Gender equity refers to fairness and justice in the distribution of benefits, power, resources and responsibilities between women and men to allow them to attain their full health potential. The concept recognizes that women and men have different needs and opportunities that impact on their health status, their access to services and their contributions to the health workforce. It acknowledges that these differences should be identified and addressed in a manner that rectifies the imbalance between the sexes.

Differences in mortality and morbidity rates between men and women are well established; however, the scale of these varies widely across the WHO European Region. It is important to look at differences in health beyond life expectancy and to consider the health that individuals experience during their lifetimes. Where healthy life years are measured, women's mortality advantage contributes to more healthy life years but their higher prevalence of disability reduces the difference. There are also documented differences between women and men in terms of the use of health care resources, exposure to risk, vulnerability and responses from the health systems *(148)*.

Men's ill health is influenced by gender roles and norms: greater levels of occupational exposure to physical and chemical hazards, risk behaviours associated with male lifestyle, and health behaviour paradigms related to masculinity (men are less likely to visit a doctor when they are ill and are less likely to report on the symptoms of disease or illness).

Gender norms and roles shape the way adolescents view sexuality and play an important role in attitudes towards risk-taking and access to and use of information and services. Women's access to sexual and reproductive health services may be limited by gender stereotypes and socioeconomic barriers to services *(91)*.

The importance of early childhood care and education is based on the assumption of a universal, high-quality, free primary and secondary education system. Most countries in the European Region have well-established systems, but in some countries girls are not equally enrolled in secondary education or have higher drop-out rates. This not only has lifelong impact on gender inequality, it also reduces countries' potential for economic development and growth.

Women are a group at risk among older people with a low socioeconomic position. Special attention should be paid to older women who, owing to a longer life and a different life-course, have more health problems in old age; in addition, they are more likely to need and not to be able to access health services.

Solutions that work

World Health Assembly resolution WHA60.25 (2007) calls for the use of sex-disaggregated data and gender analysis to inform health policies and programmes and to ensure that gender perspective is incorporated in all levels of health care delivery and services, including those for adolescents and young people *(113)*. In 2007, the European Institute for Gender Equality (EIGE) was created as a European agency that supports the EU and its Member States in their efforts to promote gender equality. Failing to address gender inequities and discrimination will compromise service efficacy and will make achieving Millennium Development Goals 4 and 5, and indeed, other Millennium Development Goals much more difficult *(55)*.

A universal, high-quality, affordable early years, education and care system is essential for gender equality, enabling women to work and contribute to family income, levelling up the life chances of children who experience other disadvantages in life (such as with disabilities or from ethnic groups such as Roma) and enabling women to be more independent in older age.

Actions across the life-course to tackle health inequities and their social determinants

Some strategies for intervention to tackle health inequities and their social determinants can be derived at key stages of the life-course.

- *Maternal and child health*. Supporting maternal and infant health requires a broad range of policies, not simply within the health sector. Important policies include a minimum standard of living; enabling reproductive choice; protecting pregnant women in the workplace; enabling mothers to return to work; supporting parents with flexible arrangements and parental leave; and promoting gender equality. Such policies require the broad involvement of government, the private sector and nongovernmental actors.
- *Children and adolescents*. The health, education, social protection and labour and employment sectors are jointly responsible for the health and development of children and adolescents. Joint working may be assisted by a framework of accountability of each sector for the health of children and adolescents and health-related issues, for example via a set of jointly owned targets and indicators, linked to financing. Developing a national health information system with well-defined indicators allows trends in the health and development of children and young people to be monitored, both for the population as a whole and across the social distribution. Reviewing the legal, policy and regulatory framework, in the context of a strategy for the health of children and adolescents, allows the necessary changes to be made to respect, protect and fulfil the rights of children and adolescents to health and their access to high-quality health services *(91,106,149)*.
- *Healthy adults*. In Europe, work plays a central role in society: it provides the means of acquiring income, prestige and a sense of worth, and it offers a way of participating and being included as a full member in the life of the community. Being unemployed effectively excludes people from this participation and the benefits that employment brings. However, levels of unemployment have risen dramatically in some parts of Europe in recent years, particularly among younger workers, as a consequence of the economic crisis.

  Every country should aspire to reduce people's exposure to unhealthy, unsafe work and strengthen measures to secure healthy workplaces. This includes improving psychosocial conditions to reduce stress, through measures such as job control, job security, flexible hours and other family-friendly practices, adequate social protection, and rewards and status commensurate with effort.

The social and economic development of society requires balanced participation of men and women in the labour market and in family life, with consequences for growth and jobs, social inclusion of vulnerable groups, reductions in child poverty and increased gender equality. Achieving these goals requires broad-ranging policies to be implemented in education, employment, health and social welfare, to give men and women real life chances and choices.

- *Healthy older people*. The promotion of healthy ageing requires action on fiscal, social welfare, health services, transport, urban planning, housing, justice and education policies. While some of these policies can only be delivered nationally, others may be achieved more easily at the local level, yet within the context of a broader national health strategy or plan *(150)*. There is also an international dimension of increasing numbers of migrant care workers, many of them in unprotected, non-recognized jobs within private households *(151)*.

  A variety of sectors can develop age-friendly policies and supportive environments to enable full participation in community life and to prevent disability. These include flexible working hours and modified working environments; urban design and road traffic measures to create streets for safe walking; exercise programmes for maintaining or regaining mobility; lifelong learning programmes; providing hearing and visual aids; cost-effective procedures such as cataract surgery and hip replacements; and schemes to enable older people to continue to earn a living.

  Other policies related to societal issues, norms and values span the life-course.

- *Migrants*. Policies that promote social inclusion may include measures to combat discrimination; educational policies that pay special attention to the needs of migrants; employment policies aimed at removing barriers in the labour market; social protection policies; housing and environmental policies to improve living conditions; and health polices to ensure equitable access to services. Equity-oriented health impact assessment can be used to review how policies across sectors affect the social determinants of health.

- *Roma*. Governments are required to adhere to and implement the commitments already made through international instruments around social inclusion, poverty, and health and discrimination. For example, the 12 countries participating in the Decade for Roma Inclusion 2005–2015 have committed to developing a national Decade action plan. Furthermore, the issues of Roma rights and inclusion will be relevant when new countries wish to join the EU.

- *Gender mainstreaming*. Actions across the life-course need to tackle the different roles and norms that society assigns to men and women from birth, and the unequal distribution of power and resources that these imply. In health, exposure to risk and vulnerability are influenced by (biological) sex and (socially constructed) gender in all countries, socioeconomic groups and ages. The systematic integration of gender considerations into planning, implementation and monitoring of policies and programmes is known as gender mainstreaming.

The voices and empowerment of people and patients

A core principle of Health 2020 is the importance of participation and responsiveness, with the full engagement of people. Empowerment is a multidimensional social process through which individuals and populations gain better understanding of and control over their lives. As part of the emancipation and literacy movement in general, people are increasingly seen as the co-producers of their own health. They need to be empowered to take control of the determinants of their own health. In addition, as patients they are becoming active and informed actors, participating in making decisions on their own treatment. Increased health literacy and access to good health-related information are prerequisites.

Increasing evidence demonstrates that health care becomes more effective if patients are more involved in the whole health care process. Patients need to be placed in the centre of that process and to participate in managing it, especially since health care itself is becoming ever more complex and personalized but also because an ageing population increasingly has multiple and chronic conditions that require the involvement of a team of health professionals. Social and geographical inequities in terms of education, employment status, access to information technology and rural living, should not impede opportunities to participate.

The WHO European Region has been at the forefront of forming innovative partnerships with civil society *(152)*, including with communities of key populations at higher risk, such as people living with HIV, and with nongovernmental organizations that advocate for and provide services. Several pan-European networks and organizations have emerged, and the number and size of networks of people living with HIV have increased *(153)*.

Civil society is a key actor in formulating, promoting and delivering change. Civil society should be considered as an equal actor in delivering health services. Civil society organizations have proven to be able to provide health services, especially to populations that would otherwise not be accessing them, because of widespread stigma and discrimination among health professionals as well as for other reasons.

People empowerment is essential for improving health and its determinants. Patient empowerment and patient-centred care are considered to be important elements for improving health outcomes, health system performance and satisfaction. Together, these processes can reduce the use of health services and health care costs, and bring about better communication between patients and health professionals and better adherence to treatment regimens. Care that is truly patient-centred improves the perception of care quality, and it can improve treatment compliance and outcomes as well as reducing unnecessary care. Patients and their families become part of the health care team in making clinical decisions. In addition, patient-centred care considers cultural traditions, personal preferences, values, family situations and lifestyles. This approach requires greater investment in patient education and health literacy – much can be done here by fostering civil society involvement.

Patients can be more involved at various levels. At a collective level, it is important that everyone can take part in the societal debate about social welfare and protection, health and health care. At a more individual level, information is provided to better enable people to take informed decisions about their health and treatment and to monitor the quality of services. This also includes increased choice of provider, public reporting of providers' outcome data and access to personal medical records.

Finally, individual patients' rights are defined and formally adopted to enforce the fundamental human rights of privacy and personal integrity in the specific context of health care. Where these patients' rights have a more preventive and sometimes a more declaratory nature, they are complemented by legal provisions on professional liability, compensation and redress to take action in case patients are harmed.

Although patients can be empowered in different ways, many barriers still need to be overcome, including cultural, social or even health care related ones. Indeed, not everyone is capable or willing to take control over his or her health and treatment. Besides, health professionals also need to be convinced and motivated to allow patients to take a leading role in their treatment.

In addition to these shifts in attitude, policy-makers face other important challenges when designing a framework for patient empowerment, including those for wider public engagement in healthy lifestyles and behaviours and patient involvement in their treatment and care. An important challenge is how to establish effective information strategies. Again, health literacy needs to be improved. Another challenge is how to strengthen consumer choice, as a way to ensure trust and self-determination, without falling into the pitfall of consumerism that, in turn, may jeopardize efforts to improve the quality of health care by making health care more evidence-informed and coordinated.

Healthy living for young people may be adopted as one of the focal areas for investing in health and empowering people. Young people themselves need to contribute to such strategies, and a broad range of stakeholders can be mobilized to support health programmes for young people. These can include peer-to-peer education, involvement of youth organizations and school-based health literacy programmes. Maintaining mental and sexual health is of particular importance.

Tackling Europe's major disease burdens

Health 2020 focuses on a set of effective integrated strategies and interventions to address major health challenges across the Region related to both noncommunicable and communicable diseases. Both areas require a combination of determined public health action and health care system interventions. The effectiveness of these is underpinned by actions on equity, the social determinants of health, empowerment and supportive environments. In particular, a combination of approaches is required to successfully address the high burden of noncommunicable diseases in the Region.

Health 2020 supports the implementation of integrated whole-of-government and whole-of-society approaches that have been agreed on in other regional and global strategies, since it is increasingly recognized that action to influence individual behaviour has limited impact. Noncommunicable diseases are unequally distributed within and between countries and are closely linked to action on the social determinants of health. In addition to the need to prevent disease, health systems face major challenges in addressing the rise in chronic diseases, including mental health problems and age-related conditions.

Noncommunicable diseases

Situation analysis

In the European Region, noncommunicable diseases account for the largest proportion of mortality, with about 80% of deaths in 2008. Among broad groups of causes, mortality (all ages) from cardiovascular diseases accounts for nearly 50% of all deaths, but this varies across the Region depending on the progress and scale of risk factor development: the figure ranges from 35% in the EU15 to 65% in the CIS countries. Cardiovascular diseases are also the most important causes of premature death in the European Region, although their levels have started to decline recently. The burden of disease resulting from musculoskeletal conditions and neurodegenerative disorders is also increasing with an ageing population.

The patterns of mortality and the burden of disease are shifting within noncommunicable diseases and relative to other disease groups within the European Region. During the past two to three decades, overall mortality from cardiovascular diseases has declined in the European Region, but some gaps have widened: mortality has been halved in the EU15 countries during that period but has increased by one tenth in CIS countries. The overall cancer mortality situation may appear to be relatively unchanged, but this masks differences, such as a steep decline in death rates from lung cancer among men but a rise of the same magnitude among women *(70)*.

Noncommunicable diseases also dominate the list of the main causes of the burden of disease in the Region, with unipolar depressive disorders and ischaemic heart disease being the leading causes of lost DALYs. Noncommunicable diseases interact with each other: mental disorders, for instance, are overrepresented among people with cardiovascular disease, cancer and diabetes mellitus. Depression adversely affects the course and outcome of chronic diseases, and, in turn, the presence of other disorders worsens the prognosis of depression *(154)*.

These diseases have a significant economic impact. For example, cardiovascular diseases cost the EU economies an estimated €192 billion per year *(155)*. Apart from growing costs to the health care system, there are broader effects. Employers carry a burden of absenteeism, decreased productivity and employee turnover, and individuals and their families face reduced income, early retirement, increased reliance on welfare support and a burden of direct and indirect health care costs *(156,157)*. The state faces huge losses in taxes, both from employment and from reduced consumer spending on items subject to tax (such as VAT).

The outlook for the burden of these main diseases is a balance of three contributory factors: demographic changes, with the ageing of populations and shifts through migration; temporal and geographical changes in modifiable risk factors linked to urbanization and economic globalization; and a relative decline in infectious diseases. Tobacco use among women and girls is increasing in the European Region, especially in the eastern part of the Region. Alcohol consumption is rising in the eastern part of the Region but is only declining slightly in the western part of the Region. Overall the prevalence of obesity and overweight is rising alarmingly among both adults and children *(70)*.

The proportion of people aged 80 years and older is projected to grow by almost 50% within the EU during the next two decades. Migration into and within the European Region is increasing; migrants frequently experience greater exposure to noncommunicable disease risk factors and have less access to social protection and health care.

Main determinants and risk factors

The determinants of health underlying these differences are complex and involve both individual and societal factors. Individual variation in susceptibility and resilience to disease is in part genetically determined. The WHO Commission on Social Determinants of Health (CSDH) attributed health inequities to the circumstances in which people are born, grow, live, work, and age (the social determinants), in addition to the health care systems put in place to deal with illness. Wide inequities in the distribution of power, money, and resources are responsible for these social determinants *(27)*.

Most serious adult diseases have long courses of development: the health effects of health-damaging behaviour and environmental hazards often do not manifest themselves until some considerable time after people have been exposed to them, usually as adults or older. For many people and groups, the interaction and accumulation of multiple disadvantages, individual choice and life circumstances result in an increased likelihood of premature death and disability. At each stage in the life-course, supportive action at both the macro and micro levels can enhance resilience, health and well-being.

Exposure to health-damaging conditions and vulnerability are unequally distributed in society according to socioeconomic position and demographic markers such as race, ethnicity or sex. For example, higher educational status is closely associated with healthier eating and less smoking. They are also significantly influenced by a consumer society, extensive marketing of products and – in many societies – a lack of regulation of harmful goods.

Evidence indicates that risk factors for noncommunicable diseases such as type 2 diabetes mellitus and heart disease start in early childhood and even earlier during fetal life. Socioeconomic status in early life greatly influences health, including noncommunicable diseases in later life. Health and activity in older age are the sum of the living conditions and actions of an individual during the whole lifespan. A life-course approach is required to reduce the human and social costs associated with the current burden of noncommunicable diseases.

Solutions that work

Prevention: determinants and risk factors

Four common lifestyle and behavioural factors need to be addressed: tobacco consumption; the harmful use of alcohol; physical inactivity; and unhealthy diets *(20,158–161)*. Although specific interventions are described below, since individuals and populations have multiple risk factors, an integrated approach combining multiple interventions, is more likely to be effective. In addition, it should be noted that there has been an increasing tendency to use regulations and restrictions where these are seen to be effective and socially acceptable (such as on tobacco).

Evidence-informed and cost-effective strategies for reducing tobacco use have been identified, comprising the WHO Framework Convention on Tobacco Control *(20)* and six MPOWER *(162)* strategies supporting the Convention at country level: monitoring tobacco consumption and the effectiveness of preventive measures; protecting people from exposure to tobacco smoke; offering assistance for smoking cessation; warning about the dangers of tobacco; enforcing restrictions on tobacco advertising, promotion and sponsorship; and raising taxes on tobacco. Tobacco control interventions are the second most effective way to spend funds to improve health, after childhood immunization. If only one article of the WHO Framework Convention on Tobacco Control can be implemented, increasing the price of tobacco through higher taxes is the single most effective way to reduce tobacco consumption and encourage tobacco users to quit *(163)*.

For reducing the harmful use of alcohol, interventions that can provide a change of context to encourage and empower people to make healthy decisions can include, at the discretion of each country: establishing a system for specific domestic taxation on alcohol accompanied by an effective enforcement system, which may take account of, as appropriate, the alcoholic content of the beverage; regulating the number of and location of on-premise and off-premise alcohol outlets; regulating the days and hours of retail sales; establishing an appropriate age for purchasing and consuming alcoholic beverages and other policies to raise barriers against sales to and consumption of alcoholic beverages by adolescents; introducing and enforcing an upper limit for blood alcohol concentration, with a reduced limit for professional drivers and young or novice drivers; promoting sobriety checkpoints and random breath-testing; supporting initiatives for screening and brief interventions for hazardous and harmful drinking in primary health care and other settings, which should include early identification and management of harmful drinking among pregnant women and women of childbearing age; and developing effective coordination of integrated and/or linked prevention, treatment and care strategies and services for alcohol-use disorders and comorbid conditions, including drug-use disorders, depression, suicide, HIV infection and TB *(164)*.

Regular physical activity provides significant benefits for health, reducing the risk of most chronic noncommunicable diseases and contributing to mental health and overall well-being *(165)*. Taking part in physical activity also increases opportunities for social interaction and feeling part of the community *(166)*. The health benefits of moderate to intense physical activity must be emphasized: adults should accumulate at least 30 minutes per day and children and adolescents at least 60 minutes per day *(167)*. If inactive or almost inactive groups were empowered to engage in some activity, this would produce the greatest health gains. Social and physical environments need to be designed so that physical activity can be safely and easily integrated into people's daily lives: for example, urban planning and integrated transport systems to promote walking and cycling *(168)*.

In order to prevent noncommunicable diseases, a healthy diet needs to aim to achieve energy balance and a healthy weight; limit energy intake from total fat and shift fat consumption away from saturated fats to unsaturated fats and towards eliminating *trans*-fatty acids; limit the intake of free sugar; limit salt (sodium) consumption from all sources and ensure that salt is iodized; and increase consumption of fruit and vegetables, legumes, whole grains and nuts. As indicated in the WHO Global Strategy on Diet, Physical Activity and Health *(169)*, countries should adopt a mix of actions in accordance with their national capabilities and epidemiological profile, including: education, communication and public awareness; adult literacy and education programmes; marketing, advertising, sponsorship and promotion; labelling; and controlling health claims and health-related messages. Further, national food and agricultural policies should be consistent with protecting and promoting public health.

In addition to health promotion and disease prevention in relation to the four main risk factors outlined above, links should be made to sexual health, infectious diseases and the environment and health, particularly for preventing cancer, as well as to medical genetics. Legislation and enforcing regulations can limit exposure to carcinogenic substances in the workplace and environment. Promoting safe sex and vaccination can prevent the transmission of viruses known to cause cancer such as human papillomavirus and hepatitis B.

The risk of a person developing diseases depends on interaction between the individual, his or her personal susceptibility and the wider environment. Many diseases, such as diabetes and asthma, have a complex pattern of inheritance *(170)*. Understanding individuals' genetic make-up may enable more personalized prevention of disease, but good evidence still needs to be gathered to demonstrate that this improves on already effective population-level prevention strategies *(171)*. In contrast, there is growing evidence about the role of environmental determinants of chronic diseases. For example, indoor and outdoor air pollution increases the risk of asthma and other respiratory diseases, and fine particulate matter in the air increases the risk of cardiovascular disease and lung cancer, significantly affecting life expectancy *(172)*. Radon is the second leading cause of lung cancer after tobacco smoking. Primary prevention of disease – avoiding its occurrence – focuses on eliminating or reducing exposure to environmental risk factors *(173)*. Declining cardiovascular mortality after smoking is banned in public places or ambient air pollution is reduced are examples of how successful actions addressing the environmental determinants of health can benefit health.

Early disease: screening and early diagnosis

The earliest possible detection of disease and the best possible integrated and multidisciplinary care are required when the disease is established and effective treatment exists. For example, about one third of people with cancer can be cured if the cancer is detected and effective treatment is started early enough. Raising awareness of the early signs and symptoms of cancer among the public and health professionals can lead to cancer being detected at earlier stages of the disease (down-staging) and more effective and simpler therapy. There are currently differences in early detection both within and between countries. Where health systems can support an organized, population-level screening programme that reaches those likely to benefit, screening can prevent disability and death and improve the quality of life. For example, evidence indicates that screening is effective for the early detection of breast and cervical cancer in countries with sufficient resources to provide appropriate treatment *(174)*.

Other evidence-based clinical preventive procedures include assessing individual people for elevated risk of cardiovascular disease using an absolute risk approach, based on variables such as age, sex, smoking history, diabetes status, blood pressure and cholesterol levels. Multidrug therapy (aspirin, ACE inhibitor, beta-blockers or diuretics, and statins) for people with an estimated overall risk of dying from a cardiovascular event exceeding 15% during the next 10 years has been shown to be very cost-effective even in low and middle income countries *(175)*.

Preventing disability

Chronic noncommunicable diseases can be major causes of disability, such as blindness and lower-limb amputation for people with diabetes or motor dysfunction following stroke. Musculoskeletal disorders are estimated to account for half of all absence from work and for 60% of permanent work capacity lost in the EU.

This is not inevitable. Prompt and effective treatment can be curative and/or reduce the chances of recurrence or long-term consequences; rehabilitation and improved models of care can shift conditions from being disabling to manageable; and adjustments to the home and work environment can keep people independent and economically active. For instance, following myocardial infarction, cardiac rehabilitation with a focus on exercise is associated with a significant reduction in mortality; and treatment of stroke through stroke unit care, for example, reduces the proportion of those dying or depending on others for their primary activities of daily living by 25%. Furthermore, although the prevalence and severity of many chronic conditions typically increase as people get older, they are not an essential consequence of ageing.

Palliative care is an integral part of long-term care, supporting people so they can achieve the best quality of life possible at the end stages of their disease and providing a peaceful and painless end to life. Most typically associated with cancer, such end-of-life care benefits people with several chronic conditions. Simple and relatively inexpensive measures such as improving access to oral morphine for adequate pain relief can improve the quality of life of many people.

Overall: an integrated approach

There were several important developments in noncommunicable diseases during 2011. The First Global Ministerial Conference on Healthy Lifestyles and Noncommunicable Disease Control took place in Moscow in April 2011 with its outcome, the Moscow Declaration *(176)*, then being endorsed by the World Health Assembly in May 2011 (177). The WHO Regional Committee for Europe endorsed action plans for both noncommunicable diseases (178) and alcohol *(179)* in September 2011. Finally, a High-level Meeting of the United Nations General Assembly on the Prevention and Control of Non-communicable Diseases was convened, linking the noncommunicable disease and development agendas. The resulting Political Declaration *(180)* outlined the magnitude, threat and impact of noncommunicable diseases, with agreement on ways to respond to the challenge through whole-of-government and whole-of society efforts.

Regional priority action areas include the United Nations 2011 Political Declaration on noncommunicable diseases *(180)*; the WHO Framework Convention on Tobacco Control *(20)*; the Global Strategy on Diet, Physical Activity and Health *(169)*; the global strategy and regional action plan on the harmful use of alcohol *(179)*; the action plan for the prevention and control of noncommunicable diseases *(178)*; and the mental health action plans. In each case, health promotion, as defined in the Ottawa Charter for Health Promotion *(30)*, is at the core. These action areas all encourage governments to develop intersectoral strategies, with goals and targets, on key challenges related to noncommunicable diseases.

Two disease groups (cardiovascular diseases and cancer) cause almost three quarters of deaths in the WHO European Region, and three main disease groups (cardiovascular diseases, cancer and mental disorders) cause more than half the burden of disease (measured using DALYs). Much premature mortality is avoidable: estimates indicate that at least 80% of all heart disease, stroke and type 2 diabetes and at least one third of cancer cases are preventable (181). Inequalities in the burden of noncommunicable diseases within and between countries demonstrate that the potential for health gain is still enormous.

The main priority is to implement effective interventions more equitably and on an appropriate scale, ensuring that existing knowledge is better and more fairly applied. Noncommunicable diseases share many common risk factors, underlying determinants and opportunities for intervention along both the course of disease and the life-course. For example, seven leading risk factors (tobacco use; alcohol consumption; high blood pressure; high cholesterol; overweight; low fruit and vegetable intake; and physical inactivity) account for almost 60% of the burden of disease in Europe. Taking an integrated and common risk factor approach to disease prevention and a chronic care approach are likely to benefit several conditions simultaneously *(182)*.

The European Strategy for the Prevention and Control of Noncommunicable Diseases *(183)* promotes a comprehensive and integrated approach to tackling noncommunicable diseases: promoting population-level health promotion and disease prevention programmes; actively targeting groups and individuals at high risk; maximizing population coverage of effective treatment and care; and integrating policy and action to reduce inequity in health. In accordance with an international focus on "best buys" *(184,185)*, the action plan for implementation of this Strategy *(178)* has focused particular attention on a set of priority interventions chosen for their potential effects on mortality and morbidity: promoting healthy consumption via fiscal and marketing policies; replacing *trans*-fatty acids in food with polyunsaturated fat; reducing salt consumption; assessing and managing cardio-metabolic risk; and early detection of cancer. These are supported by interventions to promote active mobility and promote health in settings, such as through urban design and promoting health in the workplace.

Added to this is consideration of vaccination for the vaccine-preventable types of cancer (hepatitis B for liver cancer and human papillomavirus for cervical and other types of cancer). In terms of potential effects on the quality of life, a further area deserving special mention is palliative (end-of-life) care, especially effective pain management.

Mental health

Situation analysis

Mental disorders are the second largest contributor to the burden of disease (measured using DALYs) in the European Region (at 19%) and the most important cause of disability. The ageing population leads to an increase in the prevalence of dementia. Common mental disorders (depression and anxiety) affect about 1 in 4 people in the community every year. However, about 50% of people with mental disorders do not receive any form of treatment. Stigma and discrimination are major reasons why people avoid seeking help.

Mental health is a major contributor to inequity in health in Europe. Mental health problems have serious consequences, not only for individuals and their families but also for the competitiveness of the economy and the well-being of society. Poor mental health is both a consequence and a cause of inequity, poverty and exclusion. Mental health is also a strong risk factor for morbidity and mortality from other diseases. It has been demonstrated that the presence of depression, in particular, strongly affects the survival rates of people with cardiovascular diseases and cancer. Depressive disorder is twice as common among women as among men.

Nearly all countries in the European Region have mental health policies and legislation, but the capacity and quality of services is uneven. Whereas some countries have closed or reduced the number of institutions and have replaced them with a variety of community-based services, many other countries still rely on basic and traditional psychiatric services and use up to 90% of the mental health budget on mental institutions. Investment in well-being programmes and preventing disorders in childhood, often the precursors of lifelong suffering, is negligible.

The most cost-effective intervention at the population level is creating employment, either in the public sector or by creating incentives for expanding the private sector. Of growing interest is the interface between employment and mental health, since good-quality employment is good for health and its determinants (such as a good standard of living, self-esteem, social participation). This can also contribute to a healthy and productive workforce, with secondary benefits for families and communities. Effective occupational health services can identify, monitor and support people at risk at from an early stage. For groups at higher risk, public health interventions such as screening and information can be effective. People with mental health problems need to be detected in primary care, and people with severe conditions should be referred to specialist services.

Solutions that work

A WHO European regional strategy for mental health is being developed, and it is anticipated that this will be presented to the WHO Regional Committee for Europe in 2013. Challenges for mental health include sustaining the population's well-being at times when economic growth is minimal and public expenditure is facing cuts. This may result in higher unemployment (particularly long-term unemployment) and an increase in poverty, with an associated risk of depression, while mental health services undergo budget cuts. The psychosocial stress associated with job insecurity is also considerable. A particular challenge is to promote the early diagnosis of depressed people and to prevent suicide by initiating community-based intervention programmes and services such as telephone hot lines and counselling support. Young people at risk can be helped by developments in schools such as early warning systems and anti-mobbing campaigns. Research is beginning to yield a better understanding of the damaging association between mental health problems and social marginalization, unemployment, homelessness and alcohol and other substance use disorders. New forms of addiction related to virtual worlds also need to be addressed.

Some countries are responding to the threat to people's mental health by expanding counselling services. Awareness is also growing of the association between debt and depression, and debt advice services are playing crucial roles in providing financial security.

A rights-based approach to health care requires mental health services to be safe and supportive and every patient to be treated with dignity and respect. People receiving mental health care should be involved in decision-making concerning their individual care. Mental health professionals should encourage patients to make their own choices regarding their health care, facilitated by providing appropriate information, and people who use mental health services should be involved in designing, delivering, monitoring and evaluating them.

At the population level, the threat to mental health offers opportunities to establish links between sectors that rely on each other but do not traditionally work together, such as benefit offices, debt counsellors and community mental health services. Coordination is essential for effectiveness and efficiency, and community mental health personnel are well positioned to take this role.

WHO has produced the mental health Gap Action Programme (mhGAP) *(186)*, which specifies effective interventions for mental disorders. The WHO Regional Office for Europe's forthcoming mental health strategy will address ways to improve the mental well-being of the population, prevent the development of mental disorders and offer equitable access to high-quality services. The Regional Office is also working with countries to develop a mental health workforce that is competent to face the challenges.

Mental health care systems have expanded beyond their former focus on treating and preventing disorders. Mental health policies, legislation and implementation strategies are being transformed towards creating structures and resources that aim to empower people with mental health problems to make use of their inherent potential and to participate fully in societal and family life. This task can be achieved only by providing services and activities that empower individuals as well as communities and that protect and promote human rights.

Injuries and violence

Situation analysis

Injuries, whether unintentional (from road traffic accidents, poisoning, drowning, fires and falls) or intentional (from interpersonal and self-directed violence), cause 700 000 deaths each year in the WHO European Region *(187)*. They are the leading causes of death among people aged 5–44 years. The leading causes of injury are road traffic accidents, poisoning, interpersonal violence and self-directed violence. Injuries are responsible for 9% of the deaths in the Region but for 14% of the burden of disease as measured by DALYs *(188)*. Although there has been a general downward trend, mortality rates from injuries have increased in times of socioeconomic and political transition *(189)*. Injuries are a major cause of health inequities in the Region. The mortality rates in countries that are members of the CIS are still four times higher than those in the EU, and 76% of the deaths in the Region are in low- and medium-income countries.

Within countries, injuries and violence are strongly linked to socioeconomic class and cause health inequities. There are cross-cutting risk factors for the different types of injury, such as alcohol and drug misuse, poverty, deprivation, poor educational attainment and unsafe environments *(190,191)*. These also cut across other disease areas such as noncommunicable diseases, presenting opportunities for joint action. Many of these risk factors are socially determined. Developing preventive strategies requires addressing the underlying structural factors and modifying individual and population-level risk behaviour.

Gender-based violence is one of the most sensitive indicators of gender inequity and can severely affect physical and mental health. There are no comparable data on this problem in the European Region, but surveys from several countries indicate between 10% and 60% of women have been attacked by an intimate partner.

Solutions that work

The Region has some of the safest countries in the world. If all countries were to match the lowest national mortality rates from injuries, an estimated half a million lives lost from injuries could be saved in the Region each year. Countries with low injury rates have invested in safety as a societal responsibility and have achieved this by combining legislation, enforcement, engineering and education to achieve safe environments and behaviour (such as on the roads, at home and in nightlife venues) *(190)*. These responses involve sectors other than health, and the challenge in preventing and controlling violence and injuries lies in ensuring that these responses are placed high on the agenda of policy-makers and practitioners from the health sector and other sectors *(192)*. A life-course approach is advocated, and interventions targeted early in life will lead to benefits in later years and across generations.

There is growing evidence about effective strategies to prevent injuries and violence, and many strategies have also been shown to be cost-effective, proving that investing in safety produces benefits for society at large. For example, every €1 invested in child safety seats saves €32; for motorcycle helmets the saving is €16, for smoke alarms €69, for home visiting schemes educating parents against child abuse €19, for preventive counselling by paediatricians €10 and for poison control centres €7 *(193)*. WHO has proposed 100 evidence-informed interventions, and implementing these would dramatically reduce the inequities in the burden of injuries across the Region *(194)*. These include a range of population-level and individual approaches to prevention, such as mitigating alcohol misuse (a major risk factor for injuries and violence). Interventions that are cost-effective at the population level are regulation, considering pricing policies and regulating advertising, and, at the targeted level, brief counselling by physicians. The WHO strategy is to work with Member States to advocate for implementing the 100 evidence-informed interventions, underpinned by WHO Regional Committee for Europe resolution EUR/RC55/R9 on the prevention of injuries *(195)*. Periodic surveys show that good progress is being made, although much more needs to be done.

Examples of specific areas of action include the United Nations Decade of Action for Road Safety 2011–2020, launched on 11 May 2011. Many countries in the Region have mainstreamed road safety into their national agenda. WHO is working with health ministries and other partners to try to achieve national targets, which in many countries include halving the number of road traffic deaths by 2020. To advocate for halting the cycle of violence, surveys of adverse childhood experience are being undertaken in several countries. The survey results are presented at national policy dialogues, at which interventions for child maltreatment prevention are given priority for mainstreaming into child health and development programmes. Greater action is also being sought in two other neglected areas of policy: preventing youth violence and preventing elder maltreatment.

Implementing evidence-informed interventions can reduce inequities in the burden of injuries. As noted above, WHO has proposed 100 such interventions for implementation and is monitoring this *(194)*. The challenge in preventing injuries and violence is to promote the implementation of such measures. Since some are outside the remit of the health sector, health systems need to strengthen their role as a steward for equitable prevention. This includes: advocacy and policy development, prevention and control, surveillance, research and evaluation, and providing services for the care and rehabilitation of injury victims. To assist the health sector in fulfilling these roles, capacity can be built by mainstreaming WHO's teach vip curriculum into curricula for health professionals *(196)*.

Communicable diseases

Situation analysis

Communicable diseases rank low as a cause of DALYs *(82,197)* but continue to cause significant avoidable illness and premature death throughout the European Region. Although spectacular progress has been achieved in many countries in controlling many communicable diseases such as poliomyelitis, diphtheria, malaria and the mother-to-child transmission of HIV, the European Region is experiencing serious challenges, including increases in the rates of HIV infection and TB, a resurgence of vaccine-preventable diseases and the emergence of antibiotic-resistant organisms.

With an ageing population, the European Region has a growing population at greater risk of communicable diseases such as influenza and severe complications such as septicaemia; in future, routine immunization programmes for older people may be needed.

As a centre of worldwide trade and travel, the European Region will continue to be exposed to the importation of infectious diseases from countries outside the Region, some being epidemic-prone, such as foodborne outbreaks and emerging zoonoses *(198)*. Further, with continuing conflicts and political tensions in a world in which biotechnology is becoming increasingly accessible, the deliberate use of infectious agents to cause harm cannot be ruled out.

The European Region, and particularly its growing large urban centres, will continue to attract migrant populations, and with them large pockets of poverty and groups with high levels of vulnerability and limited access to health care (such as those living in migrant hostels and other high-density accommodation). These groups will be at higher risk of diseases such as diphtheria and TB, which may spread to the general population from time to time.

In addition to general concerns about sustaining the overall progress made in the Region, the continual introduction of exotic infectious agents, many with epidemic potential, by international travellers and a global food chain further underlines the importance of remaining vigilant and committed to preventing and controlling communicable diseases.

Despite proven interventions with, in some cases, decades of evidence documenting their effectiveness, access to prevention and early treatment is often not available or underutilized, especially among socially marginalized high-risk groups. The increasing popularity of "alternative" practices, many with no proven efficacy, when coupled with a general distrust of government-supported medicine, leads some population groups, often in more affluent countries, to reject preventive services, such as vaccinations, or to treat infections with sham "medicines". These practices put those population groups, their children and those around them at greater risk of disease. All these factors, coupled with a general complacency regarding the risk posed by most infectious diseases, hamper the prevention and control of communicable diseases in the European Region *(199–201)*. This complacency exists despite the worrying emergence of pathogens resistant to antimicrobial drugs, especially to antibiotics *(202)*; the dramatic return in the European Region of vaccine-preventable diseases previously close to elimination such as measles, rubella and poliomyelitis; frequent foodborne and zoonotic outbreaks; and, in an increasingly globalized and interconnected world, the importation of epidemic-prone diseases such as severe acute respiratory syndrome (SARS) and H1N1 influenza *(203)*.

Preventable communicable diseases in the European Region also cause significant economic damage *(204)*, including substantial absenteeism caused by such diseases as seasonal influenza, and significant losses in tourism, trade and transport caused by outbreaks such as meningitis and *Escherichia coli* enteritis.

To meet these challenges, WHO works in active partnership with Member States and their government agencies and institutes and with key institutions in the European Region.[6]

The WHO European Region must remain focused on achieving regional targets related to controlling, preventing and, where possible, eliminating communicable diseases and must remain vigilant to the risk posed by communicable diseases in an ageing population that will become more and more vulnerable to severe complications of infection. Strong disease surveillance systems, strict infection control, universal access to and prudent use of antibiotics, comprehensive vaccination programmes and strengthened health systems are essential to guaranteeing the regional capacity to control and reduce the burden of communicable diseases.

Solutions that work

There are many proven, evidence-based and cost-effective interventions to combat communicable diseases. Most of the global "best buys" are in

[6] These include: the European Commission; the European Centre for Disease Prevention and Control (ECDC); the United States Centers for Disease Control and Prevention (CDC); United Nations programmes and agencies such as the United Nations Children's Fund (UNICEF), the Joint United Nations Programme on HIV/AIDS (UNAIDS), the United Nations Development Programme (UNDP), the United Nations Population Fund (UNFPA), the Food and Agricultural Organization of the United Nations (FAO) and the International Organization for Migration (IOM); multilateral organizations such as the Global Fund to Fight AIDS, Tuberculosis and Malaria and the GAVI Alliance; the World Bank; the Asian Development Bank (ADB); the OECD; the World Organization for Animal Health (OIE); and specialized WHO collaborating centres, bilateral ministries and development agencies, foundations and private international organizations, such as CARE and Project HOPE.

communicable diseases, including: vaccinating children against major childhood diseases; providing insecticide-treated bed nets, household spraying with insecticides and preventive treatment for malaria in endemic areas; ensuring universal access to TB diagnosis and DOTS-plus, and effective diagnosis and treatment of people with multidrug-resistant TB; preventing HIV transmission through condom use, antiretroviral therapy and harm reduction strategies; avoiding unsafe health care injections; and controlling health care–associated and community-acquired infections. Strong health information systems, including surveillance for early detection of outbreaks, are also crucial for identifying, planning and investing in the most appropriate health interventions.

Critical factors that affect the full implementation of interventions include: the burden of disease; cost and affordability; political commitment and public acceptance; health system capacity to absorb new products and modes of delivery; access, particularly for reaching populations at higher risk; and public demand and risk perception. For example, new vaccines, such as those that protect against cervical cancer, pneumococcal pneumonia and rotavirus diarrhoea, are expensive and may need to be evaluated against effectiveness measures such as cost per DALY averted, which will depend on the price, the burden of disease and public acceptance.

Successful interventions require cooperative and integrated efforts across many sectors, such as law enforcement, transport, water and sanitation, food and agriculture and manufacturing, if their effectiveness is to be maximized. For instance, many harm reduction programmes that involve providing opiate substitution therapy and needle and syringe exchange require appropriate legal policies and the cooperation of law enforcement agencies. Food outbreaks tied to *Escherichia coli* contamination are best prevented through adequate regulatory and monitoring capacity in the food and agriculture and in the water and sanitation sectors. Surveillance and alert and response capacity at points of entry (ports, airports and ground crossings) are essential components of the transport sector, in order to protect against the importation of diseases with outbreak potential.

Vaccine-preventable diseases and immunization

The creation of national immunization programmes several decades ago enjoyed high public acceptance and achieved great success, with coverage rates exceeding 90% for most of the routinely administered vaccines *(205)*, resulting in the certification of the Region as polio-free in 2002 and a reduction in measles cases by more than 90% since 1990. Lately, however, the public's risk perception has shifted towards the adverse events associated with vaccination, rather than the dangers of the actual disease, with consequent negative effects on disease control. Pockets of susceptible people remain despite generally high immunization coverage, and previously contained diseases have returned. For example, in 2007 the annual regional incidence of measles had dropped to an all-time low before the rate increased four-fold by 2011, with most cases occurring in the western and central parts of the Region.

Despite these challenges, routine childhood vaccines[7] remain crucial, life-saving public health tools, and several important new vaccines, such as pneumococcal and rotavirus vaccines, are being progressively introduced into the routine immunization schedules of Member States. Moreover, vaccines against cancer-causing viruses, hepatitis B and human papillomavirus bridge communicable and noncommunicable diseases *(206–209)*.

[7] For measles, rubella, mumps, poliomyelitis, diphtheria, tetanus, pertussis, hepatitis B, *Haemophilis influenzae* b and varicella.

Specific advocacy campaigns such as the annual European Immunization Week *(210)* offer countries an opportunity to launch widespread immunization campaigns and increase awareness towards the regional commitment to maintaining high immunization coverage.

Surveillance systems must be maintained and strengthened for all vaccine-preventable diseases. The WHO Regional Office for Europe has multiple disease-specific laboratory-based surveillance networks in place to detect cases, trace chains of transmission and even detect pathogens before clinical cases occur. Such systems involve clinicians, epidemiologists and networks of more than 200 fully accredited laboratories using WHO standards for case definition, surveillance protocols and laboratory methods to detect the circulation of pathogens in humans and environment, determine the origin and transmission pathways of infectious agents based on genetic data and monitor the effects of vaccination once implemented *(211)*.

The WHO Regional Office for Europe continues its work on linking disease surveillance networks and improving the timeliness and accuracy of data sharing. It has offered the Centralized Information System for Infectious Diseases (CISID) *(212)* as a service to the Member States for several years and more recently has launched the Laboratory Data Management System for the Polio Laboratory Network *(213)* to provide laboratory-related data for every case in near real time with a precision never before available. Similar platforms are under development for other Regional Office laboratory networks.

The history of smallpox eradication *(214)*, as well as recent episodes of laboratory-acquired SARS *(215)*, indicate that laboratories may become sources of infection, and laboratory biosafety and biosecurity must be priorities for the laboratory community in the European Region, especially since poliomyelitis is targeted for global eradication.

Antimicrobial resistance

Previous gains in life expectancy in the WHO European Region, caused in part by the introduction of antibiotics, are at risk today because of growing antimicrobial resistance. Life-saving antibiotics are becoming ineffective or dramatically expensive, posing serious technical and financial challenges to physicians, health systems and patients in all countries, especially resource-limited ones. This is true for drugs that treat many common bacterial infections, such as urinary tract infections and pneumonia, but it is even more striking in the treatment of TB, which increasingly faces resistance to both first- and second-line treatments (multidrug- and extensively drug-resistant TB).

Resistance has been found in 25% or more of bacterial infections in several EU countries. This has led, in the EU alone, to an estimated 25 000 extra deaths each year and additional health care and societal costs of at least €1.5 billion.

Furthermore, antibiotic-resistant bacteria easily cross borders, as shown by the well-documented international spread of bacteria containing the New Delhi metallo-beta-lactamase 1 (NDM-1) enzyme that makes them resistant to a broad range of antibiotics *(216)*, including those, such as carbapenem, already used to treat antibiotic-resistant infections. This situation is of particular concern in the absence of new classes of affordable and effective antibiotics, especially against gram-negative bacteria.

The evolution of drug-resistant organisms is a well-understood process that is accelerated by misuse (underuse and overuse) of antibiotics in human medicine and in animal agriculture. Poor infection control measures, especially within hospitals and clinics, directly contribute to spreading drug-resistant health care–associated infections.

Broad intersectoral initiatives will reduce the misuse of antibiotics and slow the development of resistance to existing drugs. Strengthened surveillance capacity will better document the extent of antibiotic resistance in the European Region. Joint work is also needed with the agriculture sector, where antibiotics used as a growth promoter in animals contribute to the evolution of resistant organisms in livestock.

The WHO Regional Director for Europe has made containing antibiotic resistance a special programme under her leadership. The strategic action plan to contain antibiotic resistance in the WHO European Region endorsed by the WHO Regional Committee for Europe in 2011 builds on interventions that, carried out together, are known to be effective *(217)*. The action plan includes seven key areas: promotion of national intersectoral coordination; strengthening of surveillance of resistance; strengthening surveillance and stewardship of drug use; expanded surveillance of antimicrobial use in the food animal industry; improved infection control and stewardship to prevent antimicrobial resistance in health care settings; more research and innovation on new drugs and technology; and stronger patient safety through greater awareness of antimicrobial use and resistance.

Importantly, studies have shown that simple infection control measures such as hand washing can significantly reduce the prevalence of antibiotic-resistant bacteria such as methicillin-resistant *Staphylococcus aureus* (MRSA), a major hospital-acquired infection.

TB In 2010, an estimated 420 000 new and relapsed cases of TB and 61 000 related deaths occurred in the European Region. The vast majority of TB, 87% of new cases and 94% of deaths, occurs in the eastern and central parts of the Region. The Region also has the lowest treatment success rate globally: initial treatment is not successful in almost one third of newly treated cases and more than half of previously treated cases. This reflects the high rate of TB drug resistance; multidrug-resistant TB has been found in 13% of newly treated cases and in 42% of those previously treated. If resistance is not contained, it may lead to the general loss of effective TB drugs and a return to the disease burden of the pre-antibiotic era.

The re-emergence of TB and the growing problem of drug-resistant TB, particularly multidrug-resistant TB, in some countries are linked to a failure of health systems to implement services that are responsive to the people who need health services. Although TB is not the exclusive preserve of any social class, the disease is often linked to poor socioeconomic conditions and other determinants, including crowded accommodation and homelessness. Similar to HIV, people who inject drugs and prisoners are at higher risk of acquiring TB, as are alcoholics and homeless people. TB and HIV infection are a deadly tandem, as TB is a leading killer among people living with HIV. It is also a challenging disease for the 9800 children with TB reported each year in the Region.

Some countries, including the Baltic countries, have demonstrated that long-term investment and a comprehensive and participatory approach enable the control of TB and multidrug-resistant TB. Universal access to high-quality diagnosis and treatment, including effective diagnosis and sustained treatment of multidrug-resistant TB cases, has been shown to be effective in many countries in the European Region, but it has yet to be implemented in all of them.

Diagnosing and treating people with multidrug-resistant TB are highly cost-effective interventions *(218)*. The WHO Regional Director for Europe has also made containing TB, and especially multidrug-resistant TB, a special programme, and in 2011 Member States endorsed a five-year consolidated action plan to prevent and combat multidrug- and extensively drug-resistant tuberculosis *(219)*. National TB action plans are being developed and implemented within this regional framework with the support of the WHO Regional Office for Europe, national and international institutions, civil society and funding agencies, especially the Global Fund to Fight AIDS, Tuberculosis and Malaria.

A rapid assessment tool has been developed to identify and overcome the key health system challenges in preventing and controlling TB, and it is likely to prove valuable in all the countries facing TB as a major public health problem. Primary health care services need to be fully involved in detecting and following up people with TB. Health funding models need to promote the rational use of hospital resources and to promote ambulatory and alternative models of care, including home-based treatment. WHO has validated and endorsed the new molecular diagnostic tests with which TB and multidrug-resistant TB can be diagnosed in less than two hours. These tests need to be introduced and scaled up in a rational manner *(220)*.

Since TB is strongly associated with poverty and poor living conditions, efforts to combat it effectively must include improving living standards and nutrition and therefore must involve other sectors.

Interventions should address the needs of special populations, including prisoners and migrants. It is important to bring services closer to the people with TB and to minimize the referral systems for TB among children and people with TB and HIV.

The WHO Regional Office for Europe and its partners have developed a minimum package for cross-border TB control and care, which highlights the necessary steps needed to achieve timely diagnosis and adequate treatment, compliance and follow-up of people with TB.

HIV infection

The rest of the world has been observing annual decreases in the number of people newly infected with HIV, but the eastern part of the WHO European Region has the fastest growing HIV epidemic in the world. The number of people living with HIV has tripled since 2000, contributing to an increase in the yearly rate of people acquiring HIV infection by almost 30% between 2004 and 2009. Elsewhere in the European Region, the HIV epidemic shows strikingly different epidemiological patterns, with the epidemic contained in the western part of the Region and at an early stage in the centre of the Region.

The burden of HIV is distributed unevenly among key population groups, being limited largely to defined populations at higher risk and affecting most severely the populations that are socially marginalized and whose behaviour is socially stigmatized or illegal.

Contributing to this epidemiological picture are health system and societal barriers to effective treatment and control. The eastern part of the Region has some of the lowest global rates of coverage of antiretroviral therapy for people who need treatment (less than 20%) *(221)*. Furthermore, within the Region, people living with HIV have been and still are denied entry into or deported from some countries because of their HIV status, which contributes to stigmatization and does not help control the epidemic. Controlling the epidemic requires addressing these barriers to universal access to HIV prevention, treatment, care and support.

The prevalence and economic burden of HIV are likely to increase as a result of increasing numbers of people acquiring infection and surviving longer through antiretroviral therapy. In the near future, HIV will rank as one of the most costly chronic diseases.

However, there are positive signs of change: for example, countries in the eastern part of the Region have shown progress in integrating HIV prevention with maternal, newborn and child health services. As a result, 93% of pregnant women who test positive for HIV in the Region receive antiretroviral prophylaxis to prevent mother-to-child transmission *(200)*.

Effective policies and interventions to respond to the HIV epidemic have been identified. There is clear demonstrated value in strengthening political mobilization and leadership and concentrating on key populations at higher risk of exposure to and transmission of HIV. These interventions include mass media and education; promoting 100% condom use among key populations at higher risk; expanding the treatment of sexually transmitted infections that are known to increase the risk of transmission of HIV; ensuring universal access to antiretroviral therapy and to HIV counselling and testing; providing antiretroviral prophylaxis as a highly effective method of preventing heterosexual transmission in discordant couples and mother-to-child transmission; and harm reduction measures (such as opioid substitution therapy and safe injection programmes, including needle and syringe programmes).

In close partnership with governments, UNAIDS, civil society and the Global Fund to Fight AIDS, Tuberculosis and Malaria, the time has come to increasingly promote linkage and integration of HIV and AIDS national programmes with broader health and development agendas. This is the aim of the European Action Plan on HIV/AIDS 2012–2015 *(222)* based on four strategic directions: optimizing HIV prevention, diagnosis, treatment, care and support outcomes; leveraging broader health outcomes through HIV responses; building strong and sustainable systems; and reducing vulnerability and the structural barriers to accessing services. The WHO Regional Committee for Europe adopted the European Action Plan on HIV/AIDS 2012–2015 *(222)* in 2011.

Prevention strategies can be adopted more widely to control the growing burden of the HIV epidemic and other chronic diseases affecting people living with HIV, and experience has shown that groups of people living with HIV, and other civil society groups, can best propose these strategies. Ways should be considered to enable such groups to have a voice in improving quality and to facilitate true participation at all levels, in order to allow targeted and effective interventions in diverse settings and contexts *(223)*.

Eliminating malaria by 2015

Spectacular progress has been made towards eliminating malaria in the European Region. Thanks to effective intervention against mosquito vectors *(224)*, autochthonous (indigenous) cases of malaria have declined from more than 90 000 cases in 1995 to less than 200 in 2010, with all cases in 2010 caused by *Plasmodium vivax*. This remarkable achievement largely resulted from the strong political commitment of the affected countries, reinforced in 2005 by the Tashkent Declaration: the Move from Malaria Control to Elimination, signed by Armenia, Azerbaijan, Georgia, Kazakhstan, Kyrgyzstan, Tajikistan, Turkey, Turkmenistan and Uzbekistan.

Eliminating malaria by 2015 is the key objective today. This can be achieved by providing insecticide-treated bed nets, household spraying with insecticides and preventive treatment for malaria in endemic areas. These efforts have led to recent successes: Turkmenistan was declared malaria-free in 2010, Armenia in 2011 and Kazakhstan in 2012, and transmission is believed to have been interrupted in Georgia. Assuming that malaria can be eliminated, preventing the re-establishment of malaria transmission will be crucial, especially in the context of climate change and the re-emergence of other mosquito-borne diseases recently observed in the southern part of the European Region, including West Nile fever, dengue and chikungunya *(225)*.

In this context, the Regional Office, the European Commission, the ECDC and the European Mosquito Control Association are working together to raise national health authorities' awareness of this new public health risk with and urge them to take appropriate control and preventive measures. Importantly, further research into vector biology is needed to make vector control in the European Region more effective, both in terms of controlling malaria and other mosquito-borne diseases and for improving the control of other vector-borne diseases such as leishmaniasis *(226)*.

Influenza and other respiratory pathogens

Influenza and other pathogens causing acute respiratory infections contribute to a high burden of disease in the European Region, both in terms of DALYs and deaths. Influenza A and B viruses cause epidemics of respiratory illness in the northern hemisphere that affect 5–15% of the population each winter, with highest attack rates generally among children younger than five years. Seasonal influenza epidemics alone lead to significant direct and indirect social and economic costs. Recent estimates are that the direct costs of clinic visits and hospitalization for seasonal influenza in the EU approach €10 billion per year *(227)*.

Pandemics caused by a new subtype of influenza A occur periodically. Although severity and impact varies and are difficult to predict in advance, the four pandemics that occurred between 1900 and 2010 all caused significant deaths and affected the health and non-health sectors. The four pandemics varied from very severe (1918) to moderately severe (1957 and 1968) to relatively mild (2009). Influenza A viruses infect a wide range of animals as well as humans, and pandemic viruses are usually of animal origin. Since 1997, avian influenza H5N1, which is highly pathogenic to poultry, has caused widespread economic losses in south-east Asia, Egypt and some European countries. Humans are also sporadically infected, with a high fatality rate (of 573 confirmed cases globally, 336 have died).

Severe disease associated with influenza occurs each year among population groups at higher risk during seasonal epidemics as well as during pandemics. Although routine monitoring of influenza in outpatient settings occurs in most countries in the European Region, routine surveillance for severe disease and deaths associated with influenza is limited; this contributes to the misconception that influenza is a relatively mild disease and precludes comparisons of severity across seasons and estimates of the severity during a pandemic.

Before the 2009 pandemic, countries in the Region invested considerably in pandemic preparedness because of the experience with SARS, the threat of avian influenza H5N1 and the entry into force of the International Health Regulations (2005). Although the 2009 pandemic caused mild disease in most cases, many people (even previously healthy individuals) experienced severe disease and death, and health care services (especially intensive care units) were stressed.

Influenza is a vaccine-preventable disease. Countries need to further develop and maintain robust programmes to increase vaccination in higher-risk groups and among health care workers (to protect themselves and their patients and influence vaccine acceptance in the general public). In support, many Member States run influenza information campaigns to raise public awareness about influenza, preventing transmission and promoting the benefits of vaccination.

People experiencing severe disease associated with influenza need access to expert care in hospitals and in equipped intensive care units. This is supported by training health care workers on the risk factors for severe disease and training them in recognizing the symptoms.

Influenza surveillance systems, monitoring outpatients and associated severe disease and mortality, are essential, allowing countries to estimate burden and mortality, and supporting their decision-making on target groups for vaccination.

Sustaining national influenza centres *(228)* by providing quality assurance programmes, training and exchange of information and best practice is crucial. Such centres can detect influenza activity in a timely manner and guide the health care system response; contribute to global surveillance and annual selections of virus strains for inclusion in influenza vaccines; and contribute to risk assessment of influenza viruses with pandemic potential.

Continued investment by Member States in pandemic preparedness planning *(229)* will facilitate the response to a future pandemic and contribute to implementation of the International Health Regulations and generic preparedness, in particular that of health care services.

Strategies to tackle health inequities and their social determinants for the major diseases

Again, group-specific strategies for interventions to tackle health inequities and their social determinants can be derived for the major groups of diseases.

Noncommunicable diseases

Preventing and controlling noncommunicable diseases require a whole-of-society response between governments, the public sector, civil society and the private sector. For wicked problems such as obesity, tackling the problem requires an approach based on systems thinking and analysis, collaboration between stakeholders inside and outside government and governance mechanisms that facilitate joint working across sectors and between levels of government *(85)*.

Within the European Region, countries already have many types of broad and issue-specific policies relating to preventing and controlling noncommunicable diseases in place, but the coordination between these may be weak, especially where these involve early intervention in the social determinants. An overarching policy framework and mechanisms such as defining shared goals and targets, common information systems, joint project implementation, common mass-media messages, joint planning and priority-setting activities can achieve a more integrated policy approach *(230)*.

Tobacco and alcohol control provide further examples of areas where collaborative and regulatory efforts are needed. The WHO Framework Convention on Tobacco Control requires governments to introduce multilevel regulations extending from the global to local levels, together with whole-of-government action on legislation, prices, access to tobacco products and an increase in nonsmoking environments. Whole-of-government interventions are also needed to control availability and to reduce alcohol consumption through prices and other mechanisms.

Modern health services need to be capable of meeting the long-term needs of people with chronic conditions. Problems of integrated and coordinated care often arise at the interface of primary and secondary care, health and social care and curative and public health services and among professional groups and specialties. These can be exacerbated by structural divisions, separate legal and financial frameworks, separate cultures and differences in governance and accountability. Structured approaches to managing these conditions are needed, with service delivery models characterized by collaboration and cooperation across boundaries and among professions, providers and institutions to focus on and benefit individuals with chronic conditions. Partnering with people with diseases, their families and caregivers can help to design more person-oriented disease pathways. Health system mechanisms, such as payment systems, need to encourage rather than discourage coordination and to facilitate continuity of care *(231)*.

Injuries and violence

Dealing with the wider societal and environmental determinants of injuries and violence also requires a whole-of-society approach. Preventing injury and violence is multisectoral, and governance mechanisms are needed for the health sector to engage with other sectors that are critical as partners in prevention, such as those responsible for justice, transport, education, finance and social welfare. This requires a whole-of-government approach and can be facilitated by United Nations General Assembly resolutions (such as those on road safety and the rights of the child). Safety has to be put at the forefront of the agenda of other sectors. The United Nations Decade of Action for Road Safety is one example in which multisectoral action has been promoted.

Communicable diseases

Today immunization reflects a problem of previous success. A combination of political and public complacency regarding the value of immunization challenges many national immunization programmes. In the absence of disease, immunization can lose priority. Political commitment at the regional, national and subnational levels is needed to reinforce positive public attitudes towards immunization, together with mobilizing the required resources.

Strengthening people-centred health systems, public health capacity and emergency preparedness, surveillance and response

Health systems

Providing high-quality care and improving health outcomes in all areas require health systems that are financially viable, fit for purpose, people-centred and evidence-informed. Well-functioning health systems improve population health outcomes, protect people from financial hardship when ill and respond to legitimate population expectations related to benefits and services. All countries have to adapt to changing demography patterns of disease, especially mental health challenges, chronic diseases and conditions related to ageing. This requires reorienting health care systems to give priority to disease prevention, foster continual quality improvement and integrate service delivery, ensure continuity of care, support self-care by patients and relocate care as close to home as is safe and cost-effective.

Health 2020 reconfirms the commitment of WHO and its Member States to ensure universal coverage, including access to high-quality and affordable care and medicines. It is vital to promote long-term sustainability and resilience to financial cycles, to contain supply-driven cost increases and to eliminate wasteful spending. Health technology assessment and quality assurance mechanisms are critically important for health system transparency and accountability and are an integral part of a patient safety culture.

The signing and formal endorsement of the Tallinn Charter: Health Systems for Health and Wealth *(24)* reflects the commitment of European Member States to strengthen health systems to meet these objectives. Health 2020 reaffirms the central tenets of the Tallinn Charter by putting forward innovative approaches that strengthen core health system functions. It renews efforts to find people-centred solutions resilient to economic downturns: provide effective and relevant population health services, ensure access to evidence-informed and patient-centred individual health services, generate high-quality health system inputs including human resources and medicines and provide effective governance arrangements.

Situation analysis

Despite diversity in the funding and organization of health systems in the European Region, they face similar challenges of providing comprehensive approaches to reducing the burden of chronic diseases and halting the growth in communicable diseases. Nevertheless, resources are limited, requiring difficult trade-offs, which become particularly acute at times of economic downturn. Health care has become more complex, with rapidly advancing technological progress, ageing populations, more informed service users and increasing cross-border movement. Health system responses to these changing trends require innovative solutions focused on the end-users (both healthy and less healthy people) that are systematically informed by sound evidence and are as resilient to economic cycles as possible.

European health systems have been adjusting to these challenges with continual reform and innovation. The WHO European Ministerial Conference on Health Systems, held in Tallinn on 25–27 June 2008, was a milestone that marked the importance that Member States placed on both improving and being accountable for the performance of their health systems. The political commitment was marked by the signing of the Tallinn Charter *(24)* and its later endorsement in a Regional Committee resolution on stewardship/governance of health systems in the WHO European Region *(232)*. Most countries have remained committed to the principles of solidarity even in the aftermath of the economic downturn, and others continue to move towards universal coverage. Value-for-money considerations have come to the fore of public policy discussions, both in response to long-term trends in ageing and the recent economic crisis. This is leading many countries to examine and adjust how they deliver services as well as their commissioning and governance arrangements.

Health policies, plans and strategies should be based on an understanding of the health needs of the population and a vision of the requisite public health and health care responses. However, weaknesses in the structure and function of service delivery in health systems in the Region undermine moves towards an evidence-informed and people-centred approach.

Modern public health concepts and approaches have not been put into practice in many countries; they lack national strategies for developing public health services, reforming outdated public health laws, and reviewing ineffective partnership mechanisms. Disease prevention, including upstream interventions in the social determinants, and health promotion are especially important elements of public health, but lack of investment and sometimes the unintended consequences of reform lead to weak infrastructure and low-quality services.

The structure of service delivery (both population and individual services) often reflects the past burden of disease and historical investment patterns, which is not conducive to people-centred 21st-century care processes for chronic illness and an ageing population. For example, public health services in many countries continue to focus on communicable diseases and have only slowly begun to integrate structures and activities for noncommunicable diseases. Specialist-driven and hospital-focused health care misses important health and welfare needs and is expensive, in contrast to systems focused on promoting health and preventing disease. Primary care continues to present challenges in many countries, with a narrow task profile, poor teamwork, limited recognition, weak links to higher levels of care and inadequate funding. These patterns often result from skewed health expenditure trends and professional power struggles that favour acute curative services and high-tech diagnostics at the expense of primary care, disease prevention, health promotion, rehabilitation and social care.

The structures and integration of processes are often poorly coordinated between public health services, and health and social care services, including health promotion, disease prevention, responding to acute illness episodes, care management and rehabilitation. There are many reasons for poor coordination, including weak health system governance and fragmented service delivery arrangements, lack of financial incentives and financial policies conducive to effective coordination of care, variation in doctors' clinical practice (both general practitioners and specialists) and lack of evidence-informed pathways for the whole continuum of a care episode or the pathways not being followed.

Commitment to improving the quality of both public health and health care services has been variable. This requires developing a culture of continual learning, removing administrative complexity, ensuring that safety is a key design element, ensuring that appropriate incentives support improvement, ensuring a culture of measurement and feedback, and implementing team-based approaches to delivery. These elements are not yet routinely present in service delivery organizations across the Region, resulting in care that is neither evidence-informed nor patient-centred.

There have been many innovations in health funding arrangements in recent years to strengthen universal coverage, but much needs to be done to eliminate catastrophic and impoverishing payments in the Region, especially for chronically ill people and vulnerable populations. Many countries have achieved universal coverage, providing reasonable levels of financial protection and access to health care for the whole population. Nevertheless, 19 million people in the Region experience out-of-pocket health expenditure that places a catastrophic burden on their household budgets, and more than 6 million people have been impoverished because of it. Further, many people with chronic diseases face severe barriers to accessing high-quality, continuous care management. Public coverage of chronic care services is far from universal in many countries. Countries differ widely in their cost-sharing requirements for health services and drugs for people with chronic diseases.

This leads to delays in seeking health care, which in turn affects treatment outcomes, especially for low-income and vulnerable people, contributing significantly to the observed health divide throughout the Region.

Moving to a more evidence-informed, population based, and people-centred approach poses significant human resource challenges. Health systems have shortages of the right people with the right skills in the right place, especially nurses and general practitioners. Joint working arrangements with other sectors are often poorly developed and lack shared objectives and budgets. The distribution of health workers is uneven, characterized by urban concentration and rural deficits. Poor working environments, lack of flexible working arrangements (with a feminization of the health workforce), including unsupportive management and insufficient social recognition, undermine the morale of health workers. The education and training of health professionals have not kept pace with the challenges facing the health system, leading to a mismatch between the competencies of graduates and the needs of service users and the population as a whole as well as a predominant orientation towards hospital-based services and a narrow technical focus without broader contextual understanding. There is limited enthusiasm for continued learning because of lack of opportunities for career development, low wages and lack of incentives. In many countries, the migration of health workers and workers leaving the public sector for the private sector severely affect the quality and accessibility of care and the capacity to engage with other sectors.

High-quality and affordable medicines are not yet systematically available in all countries, even for widely prevalent conditions such as hypertension, asthma and diabetes. Medicines are essential for preventing and treating diseases, and poor-quality medicines represent a public health hazard. Medicines are also responsible for a substantial part of health care costs: from 10–20% in EU countries to up to 40% in countries in the eastern part of the European Region. In several countries in the eastern part of the Region, ensuring regular access to high-quality, safe and affordable medicines is still a challenge because budgets are insufficient, supply systems are weak, supplies are often unregulated and out-of-pocket payments are high. Funding and regulating the supply of medicines strongly influences health outcomes and the financial protection of individual people. An important challenge for all countries is the managed introduction of new and expensive health technologies, such as pharmacotherapy, devices and procedures. This process is often not informed by evidence on the efficacy and safety of medicines and technologies and risk-sharing arrangements between regulators and pharmaceutical companies. Introducing and implementing generic substitution policies is one of the most effective cost-containment measures for low-, medium- and high-income countries.

Finally, governance needs extended partnerships and alliances to better reorient health systems towards evidence-informed and patient-centred approaches. This may include, among others, granting wider levels of decision-making to providers, enhancing the culture of performance and accountability based on high-quality and widely shared information and engaging with the population and communities in designing health care solutions. Strengthening governance at the policy, planning, purchasing and provision levels boosts rapid changes in the service delivery culture.

Solutions that work

Strengthening the performance of health systems has been high on the agenda of countries throughout the European Region, with new approaches and innovations for improving health and health equity. Improving the delivery of public health and health care services, generating key health system inputs such as human resources and medicines in higher quality, strengthening health funding arrangements and enhancing governance are key focus areas of Health 2020. This section highlights policy shifts and innovations in health systems that have been proven, or have the potential, to directly improve health outcomes and health equity. These proposed solutions are valid in a variety of health systems regardless of their form of funding (general tax revenue versus contributory), organization of service delivery (integrated versus fragmented), ownership of health care providers (public versus private) and the governance arrangements (centralized versus decentralized).

Public health services

Achieving better health outcomes in the European Region requires significantly strengthening public health functions and capacity. Although the capacity and resources invested in public health vary across the European Region, the need to invest in public health institutional arrangements and capacity-building and to strengthen health protection, health promotion and disease prevention are acknowledged as priorities. Reviewing and adapting public health acts to modernize and strengthen public health functions can be one way forward. Cooperation on global health and health challenges of a cross-border nature are increasingly important, as is the coordination within countries that have devolved and decentralized public health responsibilities.

Public health services need to be value and evidence based and inform policy-making, resource allocation and strategic development for promoting health. These services represent an investment that is both of intrinsic value and a factor contributing to economic productivity and creating wealth. This investment is a cornerstone of achieving Health 2020.

A unifying principle of public health is its essential "public" nature and the fact that it mainly focuses on the health of the whole population. Public health transcends the boundaries of the health sector, encompassing a wide range of stakeholders throughout society to address causal pathways – both the immediate causes of disease and the social determinants. However, in many countries within the European Region, a common understanding of what constitutes public health and public health services has been lacking; skills and infrastructure across the Region are patchy; and the capacity to meet contemporary public health challenges remains very limited in many countries.

In some countries, lack of political commitment has held back the development of public health. A key element in further developing public health is to integrate its principles and services more systematically into all parts of society, informing increased whole-of-society and whole-of-government working, intersectoral action, health in all policies and strengthened health systems.

Repositioning public health at the centre of improving health requires investing in public health services and seeing it as an investment in the long-term health and well-being of the population as a whole. Public health leaders must be capable of initiating and informing the policy debate at the political, professional and public levels to advocate for policies and actions to improve health. This debate will draw on a comprehensive assessment of health needs and capacity for health gain across society. It will require analysing broader strategies for health, creating innovative networks for action across many different sectors and actors, and acting as a catalyst for change.

Health promotion and disease prevention are particularly important elements of public health, and further developing primary health care provides a key strategic method for effectively delivering these services. A combination of a previous lack of investment in disease prevention and recent reforms and changes, including decentralizing and privatizing health care services, has meant that many countries lack relevant infrastructure and services. Overall, the share of health expenditure allocated to public health programmes remains relatively small across the Region.

Protecting and promoting population health inevitably reaches far beyond the effective delivery of the public health function in any single country. It involves countries working together to address problems arising from globalization, the work of other international organizations and actors, the effects on health of global economic and trade agreements and activities and the challenges associated with global communication strategies. It also involves joint working, both laterally, across sectors, and vertically, from local and community through to regional and national.

Many of the most pressing policy challenges affecting public health involve addressing complex problems such as health inequities, climate change and obesity. These wicked problems transcend the capacity of any one organization to comprehend or address. These also require joint working. There is often disagreement about the causes of such problems and a lack of certainty about the best way to tackle them. An approach based on systems thinking and analysis is required to appreciate and understand the complexity of the processes underpinning health and disease and for formulating the complex whole-of-government interventions required in response. This approach is both relevant and necessary to tackling the current and growing burden of noncommunicable diseases.

Health 2020 has been developed alongside a European Action Plan for Strengthening Public Health Services and Capacity, endorsed by the Regional Committee in 2012 *(233)*. The European Action Plan sets out the vision for public health in the 21st century and provides a framework for action.[8] Both Health 2020 and the European Action Plan call for a commitment to improving health and addressing health inequalities at the whole-of-society and whole-of-government levels, in which health improvement permeates arrangements for governance for health and in which decision-making reflects the core underlying principles of human rights, social justice, participation, partnership and sustainability. The European Action Plan takes as its starting point the Acheson definition of public health *(234)*: "Public health is the science and art of preventing disease, prolonging life and promoting health through the organized efforts of society".

The key areas of action to be addressed in the European Action Plan include sustaining and further developing and strengthening existing public health capacities and services, with the aims of improving health and tackling health inequalities through action on the social determinants of health. It is also emphasized that public health also plays a major role in supporting, developing and strengthening health systems. The health ministry leads the health system and is central to public health leadership and services. Thus, public health is also about health systems, and reciprocally, health systems can only be effective if they include a strong public health services component.

Both Health 2020 and the European Action Plan define the health system as it

[8] The European Action Plan for Strengthening Public Health Capacities and Services contains full details of the framework of action for public health development and the essential public health operations. It is considered to be one of the main and necessary pillars for implementing Health 2020.

was defined in the Tallinn Charter *(24)*:

> Within the political and institutional framework of each country, a health system is the ensemble of all public and private organizations, institutions and resources mandated to improve, maintain or restore health. Health systems encompass both personal and population services, as well as activities to influence the policies and actions of other sectors to address the social, environmental and economic determinants of health.

At the request of Member States, the WHO Regional Office for Europe led the development of the European Action Plan. It is based on 10 integrative avenues for action, supported by 10 essential public health operations developed within the Region. These form the cornerstone of a modern public health service.

The proposed essential public health operations are to become the unifying and guiding basis for the health authorities in any country in the Region to establish, monitor and evaluate strategies and actions for public health. Box 7 lists the 10 essential public health operations. Strengthening them requires mainstreaming the whole-of-government approach to improving health through health in all policies, which promotes an integrated policy response across sector and portfolio boundaries.

The European Action Plan for Strengthening Public Health Services and Capacity is supported by a review of public health services across the Region, evidence on institutional models for delivering public health services and tools and instruments for public health practice.

Individual health services: improving access and quality

There are effective interventions for strengthening the delivery of health services to improve access to high-quality, people-centred and evidence-informed care. The main challenge of reforming health care services is to refocus them around people's needs and expectations to make them more socially relevant and produce better outcomes. The themes highlighted below include moving towards people-centred services, strengthening and adequately supporting primary health care as a hub to other levels of care,

Box 7. Ten essential public health operations

1. Surveillance of population health and well-being
2. Monitoring and response to health hazards and emergencies
3. Health protection including environmental, occupational, food safety and others
4. Health promotion including action to address social determinants and health inequity
5. Disease prevention, including early detection of illness
6. Assuring governance for health and well-being
7. Assuring a sufficient and competent public health workforce
8. Assuring sustainable organizational structures and financing
9. Advocacy, communication and social mobilization for health
10. Advancing public health research to inform policy and practice

including a supportive and and well-structured hospital system, and ensuring good care coordination. These instruments are relevant in a wide range of service delivery settings, including organizations with various task profiles (public health, primary care, hospital, social care and others) and organizations with various forms of ownership (public, private for-profit and private not-for-profit).

Health care services need to become more people-centred, in order to accelerate gains in health outcomes in the era of chronic diseases. Chronic illness is long-term, requiring repeated interactions between the patient and the health system, and in most cases it progresses. The objective of modern service delivery solutions is therefore to create mechanisms that support self-management where appropriate and delivery of care as close to home as is safe and cost-effective. This will empower patients, who can then participate in decision-making about their own care and plan for this. This requires creating sources of information, decision aids and other mechanisms to support patient empowerment and decision-making. Action to build empowering services includes:

- ensuring patients' participation and feedback in designing, implementing and evaluating health policies and services;
- implementing models of partnership and shared decision-making by patients and health care providers, supported by training and skill development programmes;
- providing patients with appropriate information about treatment options and their rights;
- mapping barriers to access to information, care, rehabilitation and assistive devices for people with chronic diseases and disabilities; and
- creating ways to measure the degree to which care in organizations and systems is people-centred and publishing comparable performance indicators.

Particular attention needs to be paid to vulnerable populations, with stronger outreach programmes and new models of delivery. Mechanisms for delivering health care services often do not reach low-income and vulnerable people. For example, internal and external migrants, Roma populations, groups living in remote mountainous areas and drug users have difficulty in accessing publicly provided health services, contributing to the health divide. Ensuring that these people receive the care they need across the care continuum and the life-course calls for new approaches to service delivery through outreach programmes, instead of waiting for them to seek care in traditional service delivery settings. The public sector must continue to be an important catalyst in encouraging the development of outreach programmes by providing appropriate funding, creating enabling regulations and reward mechanisms, and entering into partnerships with key stakeholders.

Improving the quality of care requires further efforts on the provider side to ensure that patients systematically receive evidence-informed care, as well as determined efforts to reduce undue variation in health care practice. Effective and even cost-effective interventions are well known for much of the disease burden affecting the European Region. Nevertheless, studies show that many people do not receive these preventive, diagnostic, treatment and rehabilitation services. Improving the coverage of cost-effective treatments for cardiovascular diseases, diabetes, managing pregnancy and delivery, children's health, TB and mental health problems would go a long way to improve health outcomes in the European Region. Furthermore, patients often present with more than one condition, whereas guidelines are often based on single conditions. New lines of research are needed to support decision-making in the era of advanced chronic disease.

Health 2020 remains committed to a primary health care approach as a cornerstone of health systems in the 21st century. Primary health care is a key vehicle for addressing the challenges faced by health systems with well-trained general practitioners, nurses and other health personnel. It is also a key vehicle for delivering health promotion and disease prevention services and acting as a hub to link to other forms of care. A pathway of coordinated care needs to evolve, fostering a balanced system of community care, health promotion, disease prevention and management, outpatient specialist care and secondary and tertiary hospital care. In many countries, primary health care is indeed evolving to meet these increasing demands for system change, but in others it needs to be further enabled to improve performance. Essential ingredients include a good regulatory environment, management autonomy, improved funding, training of health personnel in public health, evidence-based medicine and management, and facility-based continuous quality improvement practices.

The world health report 2008 – Primary care – now more than ever (235) reaffirmed the importance of primary health care in health systems and the central commitments of the 1978 Declaration of Alma-Ata *(5)*. Global experience shows that the distinguishing features of effective, people-centred primary care include focusing attention on health needs; maintaining personal relationships through care coordinators who employ chronic care case management approaches; relying on registries and risk stratification for continuous and anticipatory care, rather than merely responding to events; taking responsibility for health and health determinants across the entire life-cycle, including managing the end of life using appropriate advanced planning; and integrating people as partners in managing their conditions. Achieving this requires not only reforming service delivery but also aligning health funding decisions to ensure the appropriate allocation of funds within the health sector, public policy reforms that secure healthier communities and engaged, participatory leadership.

For some time, there has been a growing concern that the current clinical and economic model that underpins hospitals is no longer appropriate or "fit for purpose". Too many hospitals are trying to provide too wide a range of services. Many countries respond by trying to centralize more specialist work and locate it in larger centres. At the same time, the growing number of patients with multiple conditions challenges hospitals organized along the lines of clinical "silos". Primary care requires the support of hospitals and their specialists to manage patients with chronic conditions effectively, but the incentives for hospitals often mean that this is not in their interests. Financial incentives structured by level of care and volume of activity undermine efforts to adopt care processes that are better integrated, including shrinking or down-sizing hospitals.

Close coordination needs to be ensured between primary care, home care, social care, ambulances, nongovernmental organizations and specialist care, with defined care pathways, shared record systems and other changes to support more integrated processes. This also includes solutions to properly integrate mental health services into family medicine and hospital care, in order to recognize the growing burden of illness and the increasing connection between mental and physical ill health.

Although health care has become more effective, it has also become more complex. People needing treatment now tend to be older and sicker and to have significant comorbidity, creating more pressure on health services and difficulty in setting priorities. Increasing economic pressure often leads to overloaded health care environments. In this context, it should be recognized that unexpected and unwanted adverse events can take place in any health care setting. Ten per cent of patients in the European Region experience preventable harm or adverse events in hospital, causing suffering and loss and taking a financial toll on health care systems. Safety is part of the quality agenda and a dimension of the quality culture, which encompasses developing networks of patients and providers; sharing experiences; learning from failure and risk assessment; facilitating effective evidence-informed care; monitoring improvements, and empowering and educating patients and the public as partners in the process of care.

An important supporting measure is adopting advanced information technology solutions that can provide timely access to comprehensive clinical information, so that health care professionals and service users can make the right decisions at the right time with no delays and no duplication of services or unnecessary use of inappropriate care, with the resulting public and private costs. Unfortunately, trends have been leading in the opposite direction, with different information technology solutions at the primary care and hospital levels, resulting in poor communication between them. Commitment, leadership and investment will be required to change this. As information technology progresses, issues of data privacy and protection require very careful consideration.

Complexity makes managing modern health care one of the most difficult managerial tasks in the whole economy. Nevertheless, many countries still consider investing in management a waste of resources and effort. There is more scope for significantly improving health care delivery by applying modern methods of quality improvement and management than by any clinical innovation currently in trials. Too little effort is put into ensuring that basic systems and organization are in place and function effectively.

Generating high-quality health system input

Human resources

In order to revitalize public health and transform service delivery, the education and training of health professionals needs to be rethought so as to improve the alignment between educational and health system priorities and the population's health needs. To support this transformation of service delivery towards an evidence-informed culture with strong coordination across sectors and levels of care, education and training need to reflect several specific factors: producing a more flexible multiskilled workforce to meet the challenges of changing epidemiology; joint working with other sectors on the social determinants of health; supporting team-based delivery of care; equipping personnel with improved skills; supporting patient empowerment, learning new approaches to consultation; and building leaders' capabilities at all levels in various organizations to support these changes. The ability to update their knowledge and competencies and to respond to new health challenges is a prerequisite for the health professionals of the future; this should be supported by ready access to lifelong learning opportunities.

At the policy level, greater attention needs to be paid to the future health care needs of an ageing population and their implications for the health workforce.

This includes revisiting the balance between the types of health workers trained and the new types of professionals needed at all levels of care. For example, the increasing numbers of people with multiple health conditions require more skilled generalists, even at the hospital level. The education, training and regulation of health professionals should be based on the best available evidence on the future health care needs of an ageing population.

Improving the performance of the existing health workforce is critical, as it immediately affects health service delivery and, ultimately, population health. Improving performance is also important from the perspective of efficiency, since hiring the extra personnel needed to deal with growing demand is often not affordable. The quality of services can be improved through accreditation and compliance with the appropriate national standards for educational institutions and for individual health workers in both the public and private sectors. Supportive management styles and working conditions have an empowering effect on the workforce, which in turn leads to higher morale and commitment and thus to better, more respectful and empowering relationships with patients. The clinical relationship between doctors and patients remains of crucial importance and needs to be supported as health care becomes more complex and necessarily multidisciplinary.

Performance and productivity can also be enhanced by improving the care process through lean pathways and bundles of care; establishing coherent interdisciplinary health care teams with effective management; establishing competency-based curricula, reinforced through in-service and out-of-service training; establishing enabling practice environments, including fair remuneration, appropriate incentives and access to the necessary resources; preventing professional hazards, and enhancing the role of information, feedback and appraisal.

Nurses and midwives have key and increasingly important roles to play in society's efforts to tackle the public health challenges of our time and in ensuring the continuity of care and addressing people's rights and changing needs. Nurses and midwives together form the largest group of health professionals in the Region. Because they have close contact with many people, they should be competent in the principles and practice of public health, so that they can use every opportunity to influence health outcomes, their social determinants, and the policies necessary to achieve change. This applies in particular to those who work in community settings, as well as in schools, industry, prisons and facilities for displaced people. Skills in exerting political influence, negotiating and making decisions, as well as financial, business and cultural competencies, will be an important part of the new repertoire of all nurses and midwives, thereby equipping them to work effectively and enabling them to work at all levels across all relevant sectors.

New challenges to health systems from technological advances and changing expectations require new kinds of health expertise and new professional groupings; examples here include health care managers, health economists, health-related lawyers, and high-level technicians and engineers.

Suitable policies and strategies should be adopted to attract and retain health care workers in rural and underserved areas. The specific challenges raised by migration of the health care workforce should be addressed by putting in place the necessary regulatory, governance and information mechanisms, in accordance with the provisions of the WHO Global Code of Practice on the International Recruitment of Health Personnel adopted by the Sixty-third World Health Assembly *(236)*. As stated in the Tallinn Charter *(24)*, "the international recruitment of health workers should be guided by ethical considerations and cross-country solidarity and ensured through a code of practice".

Medicines

There are several effective mechanisms to ensure the quality, efficacy and safety of medicines, including developing and implementing appropriate regulatory structures and legal frameworks; appropriate manufacturing, storage, distribution and dispensing of medicines; widely available information for health professionals and medicine users to enable them to use medicines rationally; and fair and balanced promotion and advertising of medicines aimed at rational drug use.

To improve access to life-saving medicines, a comprehensive set of policy instruments should be considered; areas to be covered include the rational selection and use of medicines; streamlined delivery systems; funding, pricing and reimbursement; and cost-containment and patent issues. Life-saving medicines are expensive in many countries in the European Region, contributing both to the observed health divide and to inequities in use. Many countries have implemented supply and cost-containment policies that aim to optimize equitable access to medicines, given constrained health system budgets. Increasing the use of generic medicines and improving the quality of generics are two of the most important policy instruments, not only for ensuring the efficient use of resources but also for reducing the health divide between higher- and lower-income countries.

Intellectual property rights granted to promote scientific innovation are one cause of the high prices of medicines. Countries should also promote research and development work on those diseases for which no good treatment is currently available. Although discussions on this topic have been ongoing for years, further support is needed for innovations against the diseases that disproportionately affect people on low incomes.

Appropriate use of medicines will enhance the quality of care and make more efficient use of scarce health care resources. WHO estimates that more than half of all medicines worldwide are prescribed, dispensed or sold inappropriately, and that half of all the people prescribed medicines fail to take them correctly. Overuse, underuse and misuse result in a waste of scarce resources, continuing health problems or adverse reactions to medicines. Increasing drug resistance is a key problem in the Region and undermines efforts to make progress in responding to TB, for example. Rational use of medicines means that conditions are diagnosed correctly, that the most appropriate medicine is prescribed and dispensed, and that the patient and the health system can afford this medicine. It also means that the patient is well informed about the medicine, understands the importance of the prescribed treatment and takes the medicine as required. Rational use of medicines requires the commitment and competence not only of doctors, nurses, pharmacists and users of medicines but also of politicians, policy-makers, user groups and professional associations. Innovative and effective strategies to improve the rational use of medicines include the use of therapeutic committees, electronic formularies and clinical guidelines, feedback of data on medicine use, the adoption of medicine information policies, the introduction of financial incentives and evaluation of health outcomes.

Pharmaceutical companies market many products and influence not only the prescribing practices of doctors but also the demand for medicines and the compliance of medicine users. This may lead to the irrational use of medicines. The promotion of medicines can also indirectly influence medical guidelines. Regulating the promotion of medicines is an enormous challenge for the European Region and one that has so far eluded a satisfactory solution in many countries. This must be a high priority, considering the increasing tension between the demand for health care services and the limited resources available. Good practices and lessons learned need to be shared widely.

Beyond medicines, the principles described above also apply to health technologies in general. Estimating needs and identifying high-priority technologies and devices (both medical equipment and a wide range of medical and care supplies) for health care in various settings, including the home, are significant challenges in the Region. The market value of devices for medical and care purposes is estimated to be as large as that for medicines. Managing the introduction of new health technologies is as important as it is for medicines, to ensure the efficient use of resources and equal access. This requires quality assurance of devices and services, transparent procurement procedures, management of devices both in health facilities and in home care, development of harmonized indicators for rational use of health technologies, and assessment of the implications of their use for health outcomes in a long-term perspective.

Strengthening health financing arrangements

Better health financing arrangements can address these problems and will thus improve equity and solidarity as well as health outcomes across the Region.

Achieving and maintaining universal coverage remains high on the agenda in the European Region, especially in the aftermath of the economic downturn. *The world health report 2010 – Health systems financing: the path to universal coverage (237)* provides a comprehensive overview of the global situation of universal coverage and offers actionable recommendations on how to move forward in strengthening Member States' health financing systems. Universal coverage can be approached or maintained through one, or a combination, of the following policies: increasing public funding for health through general taxes and/or a payroll tax; reducing fragmentation in the health system's funding channels (pooling); adopting purchasing mechanisms that incentivize efficient behaviour among providers; reducing inefficiency in the structure of service delivery systems; and implementing pricing and regulatory mechanisms to control the growth in the price of medicines *(235)*. Universal coverage is a cornerstone of solidarity and equity in health systems and a key instrument for delivering on the commitments in the Tallinn Charter *(24)*.

Recent experiences in reforming health financing show that moving away from broad classifications of health systems, or labels such as the Beveridge, Bismarckian and Semashko models, enables increased innovation and experimentation. For example, the boundaries between social insurance systems financed through general taxes and payroll taxes are becoming blurred, as countries are increasingly realizing that a mixed revenue base is most conducive to achieving high levels of coverage in a sustainable manner without unduly burdening the economy *(238)*. This is the frontier in health financing in terms of moving towards and maintaining universal coverage, where resources are allocated across the social distribution according to need, so as to optimize outcomes most effectively, especially in response to economic downturns.

Well-tested financial instruments are available for health care purchasers to influence and measure the behaviour of health service providers and encourage evidence-informed clinical behaviour. These instruments improve the quality of care by reducing variations in practice, inappropriate utilization and health care errors, all of which contribute greatly to the health divide that exists between countries in the European Region. In addition, paying for results defined and measured in terms of health gain could help orient health care providers towards improving health. In particular, purchasing mechanisms should be developed that support and strengthen efforts to enhance care coordination. Non-financial instruments are equally important for encouraging providers to become more oriented towards evidence-informed health care. These include professional recognition, development opportunities and performance-oriented peer culture and working environments.

There are health financing solutions that ensure a stable revenue flow to health during economic cycles. Lessons learned during the recent financial crisis and economic downturn can help policy-makers to respond better to future crises with effective policy instruments that maintain universal coverage and prepare for times when public budgets come under even greater pressure. It may not be possible completely to prevent economic downturns and their adverse effects on health and social budgets, but vulnerability to these shocks can be reduced. Countries that accumulate reserves during economic growth, or at least reduce budget deficits and external debt, can opt for borrowing or depleting reserves when the economy performs poorly. Even when these options are not available, countries can decide to give higher priority to health within the available government budget and thereby to reduce the adverse effects of the economic downturn. However, this is politically more difficult to implement.

A commitment to addressing inefficiency in the health sector is vitally important in order to secure popular and political support for moving towards and maintaining universal coverage, especially during an economic downturn. Advocating for more public spending on health is difficult when the system displays inefficiency and waste. Budget cuts create huge pressure on service providers to exploit efficiency reserves, but there is a limit to how much and how rapidly efficiency gains can help deal with economic recession, and the transition to a new, lower-cost delivery system needs to be carefully managed. Short-term solutions are important to keep the system running during a crisis, but such balancing acts may not be sustainable in the long term. For example, delaying investment and maintenance may provide temporary relief for the budget, but sustainable efficiency gains should also be sought through measures such as improving energy efficiency, shifting more care to outpatient settings, allocating more resources to primary care and cost-effective public health programmes, cutting the least cost-effective services and improving the rational use of medicines, to name a few.

Financial sustainability should not be seen as a policy objective worth pursuing for its own sake *(239)*. Fiscal constraints need to be respected while pursuing the goals of equity, financial protection and health gain. Economic policy imperatives, such as the drive for greater competitiveness, must also be seen not simply as ends in themselves but as the means to improve well-being among people in the European Region

Enhancing the governance of health systems

Good governance strengthens health systems by improving performance, accountability and transparency. A cornerstone of health system governance in the 21st century is to make health policies more evidence-informed, intersectoral and participatory, and to transform leadership accordingly. Most health policies have been developed using top-down approaches. However, in a whole-of-government environment, horizontal relationships across the whole of government need to be encouraged. Greater participation of citizens and civil society would enhance the orientation of new national health plans and strategies towards citizens and the users of health services and would articulate social values.

Applying systems thinking to the design of national and subnational health plans, policies and strategies ensures a comprehensive and structured approach to long-term planning and priority-setting. Through such means, the chosen objectives for the health system, based on social values, are well aligned with the instruments used to strengthen health systems. Health policy challenges (such as the current epidemic of chronic illnesses) are increasingly recognized as complex problems, involving large numbers of variables, many causal links and positive and negative feedback loops. Only a long-term, comprehensive and targeted approach will stem the rising prevalence of chronic disease. Monitoring and evaluation should form an integral part of policy implementation, to ensure learning and adaptation.

Health ministries and their partners at the finance, environment and education ministries need to be better empowered to make the case and advocate for investing in health and its social determinants. Evidence abounds that health contributes to greater social and economic well-being for the entire society. Nevertheless, health and policies that can improve it are often given low priority, intentionally or unintentionally, during the budget negotiation process, especially if health policy-makers do not make convincing arguments. Importantly, health systems need to function as efficiently as possible in the face of increasing demand, and health ministries should take the lead in ensuring and demonstrating the value that investment in the health system produces. Finally, the capacity of health ministries to set priorities for resource allocation decisions also needs to be enhanced, especially during economic downturns, to secure universal access to the provision of health care that is needs-driven and where low-income and vulnerable people are protected.

The new generation of health system reforms calls for an enabling environment in which partnerships can thrive, civil society can participate in priority-setting and decision-making, and individuals can take better care of their own health. Beyond public-public ones, partnerships can take a multitude of forms, such as public-private partnerships, with some services outsourced to private organizations; public funding for private not-for-profit outreach workers; private health organizations with administrative boards that include local politicians; private health organizations owned by charitable organizations; and public health organizations managed by private entities. Achieving greater diversity in relationships requires that regulatory and institutional frameworks become more open and flexible to support the formation of partnerships. At the same time, health ministries need to improve their stewardship role and ensure that the actions of all their constituents, whether public or private, are in concert and working towards improving the health and welfare of the population.

Governments have been increasingly embarking on public–private partnerships, including in the health sector, to produce desired public policy outcomes through public-private risk-sharing arrangements. Such arrangements have several assumed benefits, including additional stable capital financing when public capital is in short supply or fluctuates severely with economic cycles, more efficient resource use and a greater focus on end-user quality. Although these benefits are claimed to outweigh the additional costs of private capital, the evidence is not yet comprehensive or uncontested. An important emerging lesson is that, as a public policy instrument, public-private partnerships require diligent governance by the public sector to realize efficiency and quality gains and to protect equitable access, rather than dissipating the gains in inappropriate behaviour. All the evidence suggests that managing public-private partnerships is demanding. Overall, a well-designed public governance and accountability scheme needs to be in place, to ensure that these approaches support and deliver publicly defined goals and contribute to public value. In addition, a well-designed failure regime needs to be in place, so that the public and private sectors share the costs of failure as they do the benefits of success.

Much remains to be done to ensure that evidence is systematically used in developing and implementing policy. This requires continually disseminating new knowledge, building the capacity of policy-makers and policy analysts, and implementing sustainable institutional solutions that link the demand for and supply of evidence in a mutually beneficial, respectful working relationship. Knowledge brokerage, creative forums for knowledge translation and co-production of knowledge are key to strengthening the link between evidence and policy and to reducing the divide between those who produce evidence and those who use it. A particularly useful approach is regularly assessing health system performance. Well-developed approaches measure the attainment of health system goals based on health system strategies. Performance assessment should feed the policy dialogue within the government and between programmes, public authorities at the national, subnational and local levels, health care providers and citizens. Performance assessment is a key instrument for strengthening governance and contributes towards increased accountability.

Health security, the International Health Regulations, emergency preparedness and response to public health emergencies

Situation analysis

The WHO European Region is exposed to significant health security threats associated with emerging diseases, infectious disease outbreaks and epidemics, and natural and human-made (technological) disasters and conflicts, including armed conflicts, linked to its cultural differences or disputed territories. Natural or human-made disasters include biological, chemical and radionuclear disasters. In addition, the Region faces challenges from climate change, with increased frequency and severity of extreme weather events, continuing urbanization, growing hubs for international air travel and an increasing number of mass-gathering events.

Social diversity and inequitable access to health care also challenge preparedness efforts, leaving some populations much more vulnerable to public health emergencies. The effects of economic crises worsen this situation. Lastly, although the risk of accidental release of biological, chemical or radionuclear material is increasingly being reduced by improving safety rules and procedures, the deliberate release of such material is an increasing concern, given the easier access to sensitive information and increasingly powerful technology.

Evidence from past events indicates that weak and unprepared health systems hamper the timely and effective management of health crises and increase the risk of international consequences. The considerable investment that Member States made in pandemic preparedness before the 2009 pandemic was critical in the response *(229)*. However, in general the world is ill-prepared to respond to a global, sustained, public health emergency. Many countries in the Region need further support with strengthening their core capacity to detect and respond to potential public health threats.

Solutions that work

Developing adaptive policies, resilient structures and the foresight effectively to anticipate and deal with emergencies is crucial. The International Health Regulations (2005) entered into force on 15 June 2007 and provide an international legal and operational framework for signatories to better protect the health of their populations. The International Health Regulations specifically require all Member States to develop core capacity for surveillance and response, in order to detect, assess and report in a timely manner events involving disease or death above expected levels that may constitute a public health emergency of international concern. Countries should also have the capacity to rapidly share and access relevant information and implement WHO recommendations in the context of a coordinated international response.

As the lead agency of the Global Health Cluster set up by the United Nations Inter-Agency Standing Committee, WHO has a unique international mandate within the international humanitarian system that is also followed in the WHO Regional Office for Europe's public health emergency procedures and the day-to-day operations of the Regional Office's Emergency Operations Centre. Further, the Regional Office actively supports European Member States in strengthening their capacity to respond to all types of public health emergencies, and it plays a central role in regional and global information exchange and response coordination.

Strengthening governance, implementing emergency preparedness planning as a continuous process in an all-hazard approach, establishing sustainable crisis management and health-risk management programmes in health ministries and enhancing multisectoral coordination are effective strategies for preventing and mitigating future health crises.

Because health security challenges are complex, an effective response requires transparent and timely sharing of information and data between WHO and its Member States and the close collaboration of governments, international organizations, civil society, the private sector and other partners *(240)*. In this context, WHO collaborates closely with the ECDC and the European Commission to enhance health security at the pan-European level.

In collaboration with partners and institutions, WHO has established mechanisms, such as the Global Outbreak Alert and Response Network (GOARN), to rapidly mobilize the most relevant international expertise to respond to emergencies and communicable disease outbreaks. WHO collaborating centres, such as the United States Centers for Disease Control and Prevention's Global Disease Detection Program, (which has a hub in Kazakhstan), support the implementation of the International Health Regulations.

In the field of biosafety and biosecurity, new actors, such as the security sector, are investing in public health infrastructure and developing human resources, particularly in laboratory and epidemiology capacity in countries in the eastern part of the European Region. Such investment is in accordance with the intersectoral investment for improved health security promoted by international diplomacy through, for example, the Biological Weapons Convention, the United Nations High-Level Panel on Threats, Challenges and Change, or the EU Health Security Committee.

Further evidence needs to be compiled and applied in order to involve all government sectors, such as agriculture, transport and defence, as well as relevant communities and civil society more fully in emergency preparedness and response efforts. Emergency preparedness plans must include exercises and drills to regularly test the actual level of preparedness.

Strengthened, well-prepared and well-managed capacities to prevent and respond to health crises are legally binding requirements under the International Health Regulations. Assessment tools *(241)* help countries to evaluate their own systems and identify strengths and weaknesses. The Safer Hospitals Initiative is a concrete example of the promotion of measures to reduce the vulnerability of health facilities and to ensure that they remain fully functional in times of public health crisis. Initiatives to enhance multisectoral coordination and interdisciplinary approaches are central to improve the prevention, early detection and timely management of events and should be further strengthened during international mass gatherings. Improved alert and response systems and effective emergency preparedness can trigger significant improvements in the health system and give all actors, including civil society, a unique opportunity for recognizing their respective role and responsibility in improving the health of the population.

Good governance is essential to promote emergency preparedness, particularly through improved transparency and multisectoral coordination. Transparent and timely information-sharing must continue to improve, within countries, with particular attention to federal structures, and between countries and WHO according to the procedures of the International Health Regulations and the central role of the national International Health Regulations focal points.

New partnerships will be developed, particularly with regional institutions, in order to achieve a better geographical balance of technical partners across the WHO European Region. Greater involvement of regional institutions in networks such as GOARN will be essential, to ensure both technical expertise and cultural understanding.

Closer collaboration with EU institutions such as the European Commission's Health Threats Unit and ECDC will continue, particularly in support of the EU Health Security Initiative. This includes, where possible, further developing joint reporting tools and procedures, field missions and reports. This will allow for single reporting by countries to both WHO and the EU, the sharing of expertise and risk assessment, and the avoidance of conflicting messages in risk communication.

Creating resilient communities and supportive environments for health

People's health chances are closely linked to the conditions in which they are born, grow, work and age. Systematic assessment of the health effects of a rapidly changing environment, especially in the areas of technology, work, energy production and urbanization, is essential and must be followed by action to ensure positive benefits to health. Resilient and empowered communities respond proactively to new or adverse situations, prepare for economic, social and environmental change and cope better with crisis and hardship. Communities that remain disadvantaged and disempowered have disproportionately poor outcomes, in terms of both health and other social determinants such as education and crime.

Collaboration between the environment sector and the health sector is crucially important to protect human health from the risks of a hazardous, contaminated or unsustainable physical environment. Hazards in the environment are a major determinant of health, for both current and future generations: many health conditions are linked to the environment (for instance, through exposure to air pollution and the impact of climate change), and they interact with social determinants of health. The benefits to health of a low-carbon economy and the health co-benefits of environmental policies are being considered in the context of Rio +20 – the United Nations Conference on Sustainable Development. Countries have begun to develop policies that benefit both the health of the planet and the health of people, and they recognize that collaboration between sectors is crucial to protect human health from the risks of a hazardous or contaminated environment.

The physical environment

Most European countries saw their ranking on the Human Development Index (HDI) stagnate or decrease in the period 2005–2011 *(242)*. Lower levels of human development are associated with lower levels of environmental performance and a greater burden of environmental disease.

In the WHO European Region, environment-associated diseases cause one in five deaths. The environmental burden of ill health varies significantly across the Region, however, ranging from 14% to 54% *(243)*. Examples include the following.

- Exposure to particulate matter reduces the life expectancy of every person by an average of almost 1 year, mostly because of an increased risk of cardiovascular and respiratory diseases and lung cancer *(244)*.
- Indoor air pollution from biological agents in indoor air related to damp and mould increases the risk of respiratory disease by 50% *(245)*.
- Environmental noise causes the loss of 2 million to 3 million DALYs through increases in ischaemic heart diseases, cognitive impairment of children, sleep disturbance, tinnitus and annoyance *(246)*.
- Poorly designed and badly integrated transport systems lead directly to increased road traffic injuries and deaths, and indirectly to lower levels of active travel and greater social isolation.
- Cases of important waterborne diseases, such as cryptosporidiosis, campylobacteriosis, giardiasis and legionellosis, tripled between 2000 and 2010. Helminths affect an estimated 1 million preschool children and more than 3 million school-aged children in the European Region, reflecting the need for the provision of basic hygiene, water supply and sanitation in dwellings and other child-intensive environments *(247)*.
- Although classic water-related diseases with high epidemic potential, such as cholera, typhoid, shigellosis and enterohaemorrhagic *Escherichia coli*, are in decline in the European Region, 4 million people in urban areas and 14.8 million in rural areas still use unimproved water sources, and 34.6 million have unimproved sanitation. About 10% of the rural population depends on small-scale systems for water supply such as private wells, and these are often weakly regulated and vulnerable to contamination *(248)*.
- Within countries, people with low income can be exposed to environmental risks five times more often than their higher-income peers *(249)*.

Achieving better health and well-being requires greater emphasis to be placed on reducing environmental exposure, risks and effects while increasing equity and strengthening health governance. Reducing hazards related to air, water, chemical, food and noise pollution, achieving universal access to safe water and adequate sanitation, safeguarding drinking-water quality and promoting basic hygiene could prevent more than one fifth of the total burden of disease, and a large proportion of childhood deaths, in the European Region.

However, addressing individual environmental exposures and risks is not sufficient. What is actually required to effectively address the enormous burden of chronic diseases in modern societies is an ecological public health approach recognizing complex interactions between biological, behavioural, environmental and social factors and pursuing public health solutions that are coordinated with the pursuit of planetary economic and societal sustainability *(250,251)*.

Socioeconomic inequities and the current global economic downturn hamper progress in reducing environment and health risks. In all countries, irrespective of national income, people with a low income are much more at risk from unhealthy environments than those with a higher income. Social determinants play a significant role in the levels of exposure to environmental factors and the severity of effects on the health of individuals and populations. For example, high or growing poverty levels weaken the protective functions of the water supply and sanitation sector within national health systems. People with a low income tend to live in less sanitary conditions, in less safe neighbourhoods, closer to sources of industrial pollution and other sources of chemical and other types of contamination and in low-quality housing, and they have less access to spaces promoting healthy living *(249)*.

Water quality is under constant pressure, and safeguarding it is important for the drinking-water supply, food production and recreational water use. In the EU, the legal requirements are based on the WHO guidelines for drinking-water quality, and frequent non-compliance is observed for enterococci, arsenic, lead, nickel, nitrate and other pollutants; in the eastern part of the European Region, the level of non-compliance is higher and more pathogens are present in the drinking-water supply systems. Additional pressure is expected from climate change, population growth, industrial needs and water abstraction by the domestic sector: total water abstraction is expected to decline by more than 10% between 2000 and 2030 in the EU and create water stress in central and southern Europe and central Asia *(252)*.

Foodborne diseases are a growing public health problem, as the amount of food prepared outside the home has increased steeply in recent years. Ensuring safety throughout the increasingly complex food chain requires collaboration between the health sector, agriculture, food transport, food service establishments and the food industry. Food safety and security depend strongly on the availability of safe water, land-use policies and the availability of technological advances for improving food production, storage, transport and preparation.

Global environmental changes, such as ozone depletion, climate change, biodiversity loss, the increasing numbers of environment and weather emergencies, and the rapid introduction of new materials and technologies can introduce new health problems, amplify existing ones and highlight the weaknesses of current health systems. For example, in the European Region, some of the effects of climate change are already being felt: the 70 000 deaths in the 2003 heat-wave provided a "wake-up call" as to what could happen if no action is taken. Even greater health risks from climate change are foreseen for the future: more heat-waves, droughts, floods and fires; rising sea levels, with consequences for coastal areas and settlements; permafrost melting in the north, with risks to infrastructure and viability; and worsening of the classic environmental and social determinants of health (such as air quality, water and food quality and quantity). Changes in the geographical distribution of infectious diseases, with possible localized outbreaks of new or re-emerging infectious diseases (such as dengue), are also anticipated *(253)*. Many effects of climate change can be felt far beyond the locations in which they originally occur. They can also create conflicts and competition for resources, as well as migration. The estimated costs of economic damage are huge and range between 5% and 10% of GDP *(254)*.

Although environment and health interventions involve a wide range of actors, the various types of environmental exposure (such as through air, water, soil, food, noise and ionizing and non-ionizing radiation) should be seen as integrated determinants of health and well-being across the life-course and settings of living. Sectors such as transport, water management, sanitation, energy production and agriculture play a more significant role in influencing health than the health sector alone, and intersectoral policies work on all levels, from the local to the international. The health sector has a distinctive role of promoting public health interventions by other sectors, identifying the risks to and determinants of health, and monitoring and evaluating the effects of policies and interventions.

The countries in the European Region launched the European environment and health process 20 years ago. This process is an example of a unique governance mechanism, operating through a series of ministerial conferences, that involves ministries responsible for health and the environment on an equal footing, amplifies the links and synergy with a number of multilateral environmental agreements and enhances the partnership with other intergovernmental bodies, such as the United Nations Economic Commission for Europe, the United Nations Environment Programme and the European Commission, as well as with civil society organizations *(255)*.

Implementation of the Commitment to Act adopted by the Fifth Ministerial Conference on Environment and Health, held in Parma, Italy in 2010, will be essential to better link health and sustainable development *(256)*. In particular, the Parma Declaration set out the following environment and health priority goals, with time-bound targets to be achieved by 2020 by European Member States:

- ensuring public health by improving access to safe water and sanitation;
- addressing obesity and injuries through safe environments, physical activity and healthy diet;
- preventing disease through improved outdoor and indoor air quality; and
- preventing disease arising from the chemical, biological and physical environment.

In addition, the Commitment to Act calls for:

- integrating health issues in all climate change mitigation and adaptation measures, policies and strategies;
- strengthening health, social welfare and environmental systems and services to improve their response to the effects of climate change in a timely manner;
- developing early warning, surveillance and preparedness systems for extreme weather events and disease outbreaks;
- developing educational and public awareness programmes;
- increasing the health sector's contribution to reducing greenhouse-gas emissions; and
- encouraging research and development.

The core work of WHO, especially on strengthening national health sectors to improve national surveillance, alert and response systems, remains essential in the fight against water- and food-related diseases, as does its work on vaccine-preventable and neglected diseases. Important health gains could be obtained by more closely adhering to the WHO recommendations on vaccine-preventable diseases such as viral hepatitis A.

Health impact assessment of the environmental determinants of health and of policies across sectors is a core function of the health sector: identifying the risks, understanding how they are related to human health and developing effective and efficient measures to address them. Health impact assessment has been essential for developing and implementing environmental standards and reducing or eliminating environmental risks and exposure.

As part of the primary prevention of diseases, efforts to improve urban planning, to enable increased physical activity and to enhance the mobility of ageing populations or people with disabilities lead to better health and well-being. Safer workplaces, public places and improved housing standards reduce the number of injuries and people's exposure to environment and health risks from heat and cold and to chemicals and noise. Comprehensive systems approaches to road traffic, which improve the safety of the road environment, vehicles and drivers' behaviour by addressing the leading risk factors for road traffic injuries, such as speed, drink-driving and inadequate use of protective devices, significantly improve road safety for drivers and for pedestrians, greatly reducing the numbers of deaths and injuries associated with transport. Fiscal measures, such as pricing water and sanitation services, taxing emissions of pollutants (including greenhouse gases) and providing incentives to reorient consumption patterns, promote cleaner technologies and more rational use of natural resources and conserve biodiversity. These are needed not only to ensure better health for existing populations but also to protect future generations.

In recent decades, a combination of voluntary action and of legally binding multilateral agreements and conventions has proven to be an effective mechanism for steering policy action to address environmental health challenges. For example, the Protocol on Water and Health to the 1992 Convention on the Protection and Use of Transboundary Watercourses and International Lakes has required countries in the European Region to set targets and report progress on provision of access to water and sanitation, reduction of water-related diseases and protection of aquatic resources *(257)*. The Barcelona Convention for the Protection of the Marine Environment and the Coastal Region of the Mediterranean has had major effects in developing health-protecting measures by calling for the safe treatment of wastewater and its reuse as irrigation water (designed as a measure to adapt to climate change).

Other important examples of collaboration between WHO and other United Nations agencies on the implementation of multilateral environmental agreements include the contribution of the WHO air quality guidelines to implementation of the Convention on Long-Range Transboundary Air Pollution, and the collaboration between WHO and the United Nations Economic Commission for Europe in implementing the Transport, Health and Environment Pan-European Programme (THE PEP), a unique platform that brings together ministries responsible for transport, environment and health to achieve healthy and sustainable transport patterns. The WHO Regional Office for Europe also contributes to global conventions, such as by analysing health effects and promoting health in the Rio Conventions (in particular those on climate change and biodiversity).

The Regional Office has an important advisory and supportive role to play

[9] Halving, by 2015, the proportion of the population without sustainable access to safe drinking-water and basic sanitation.

in cooperation with other agencies of the United Nations system, such as UNICEF in the Joint Monitoring Programme for Water Supply and Sanitation to monitor progress towards Millennium Development Goal 7;[9] UN-Water (an interagency mechanism) in the Global Annual Assessment on Sanitation and Drinking-water, and the United Nations Economic Commission for Europe in ensuring equity in access to safe water and improved sanitation.

A well-functioning system of environment and health governance at the level of the WHO European Region plays a major role in bringing together stakeholders from across the sectors and stimulating coordinated action to address the environmental burden of disease. The role of civil society groups is likely to be a particularly important factor in environment and health governance in the future. In many places, political concern for environment and health is a belated reaction to pressures from civil society.

Just as the quality of the environment and the nature of development are major determinants of health, so is health an important stimulus to other aspects of development. Human health depends on society's capacity to manage the interaction between human activities and the environment in ways that safeguard and promote health but do not threaten the integrity of the natural systems on which the environment depends.

Sustainable development

The goal of sustainable development is to meet the needs of the present without compromising the ability of future generations to meet their own needs. The concept of sustainable development encompasses more than sustainability. Sustainable development implies a paradigm shift from a model of development based on inequity and exploitation of resources to one that requires new forms of responsibility, solidarity and accountability, not only at national level but also globally and across generations.

The links between better health, the economy and the environmental sustainability are well established: people who are healthy are better able to learn, to earn and to contribute positively to the societies in which they live. Conversely, a healthy environment is a prerequisite for good health *(258)*.

The global plan of action agreed at the United Nations Conference on Environment and Development in 1992 *(259)* and the Rio Declaration on Environment and Development *(260)* are still valid. However, although the WHO European Region has witnessed strong economic growth and significant progress in health, including progress towards attaining several of the Millennium Development Goals, these positive trends have been accompanied by increasing disparities, health inequity, environmental deterioration, climate change and recurrent economic, financial, energy and food crises *(261)*. The need for a new, more coherent approach to environmental policy is also illustrated by the fact that, 20 years after the first Rio summit, the key decisions in many countries that affect the environment – policies on development, urban planning, transport, energy and agriculture choices and housing development – create rather than reduce air pollution, noise, chemical pollution and traffic injuries.

Several national and local case studies have illustrated the fact that the policies of various sectors and settings can also promote health benefits. Many of them use green-economy approaches. The following examples link decisions in one area (such as transport or urban planning) with better health and well-being.

The United Nations *(262)* has argued that systemic changes are barely possible without real action to address levels of consumerism and resource use.

However, if action is taken to reduce the excessive consumption of energy, limit the use of some hazardous substances and promote changes in consumption patterns, for example, the result would be to reduce noncommunicable diseases such as type 2 diabetes and cardiovascular diseases. Healthy diets that reduce overall energy intake could not only improve health and reduce obesity but also improve the environment by reducing transport and greenhouse gas emissions. Reducing the consumption of animal fat and protein would further increase the benefits, given the land, water and energy required for their production. Much work is going into finding ways to promote healthy diets, making them the easy and popular choice and enhancing public understanding of them. Policy-makers in the Region are supported by some mechanisms and internationally agreed plans to reduce the consumption of *trans*-fatty acids and salt, such as the action plan for implementation of the European Strategy for the Prevention and Control of Noncommunicable Diseases 2012–2016 *(178)*.

One key area for action is promoting active mobility and public transport. There are numerous examples of how public transport, in combination with cycling and walking, can reduce air pollution, noise and greenhouse gas emissions, energy consumption and congestion, improve road safety and better protect landscapes and urban cohesion, while providing more opportunities to be physically active *(263)*.

In turn, these policies reduce the risk of cardiovascular and respiratory diseases, type 2 diabetes, some forms of cancer and hypertension, as well as road traffic injuries. Only recently did evidence begin to emerge that this mix of transport policies can also provide opportunities to create new jobs or to "green" existing jobs.

Great health benefits can be achieved in the housing and construction sector through a mix of measures, including: more effective use of active and passive natural ventilation for cooling; measures to reduce mould and damp; energy-efficient home heating, appliances and cooking; providing safe drinking-water; and improved sanitation and stronger buildings. Many countries, regions and cities are experimenting with cost-effective, healthy strategies for mitigating climate change in the housing sector; these should be systematically studied and evaluated for their health benefits *(264)*.

Green spaces in urban areas positively affect health. Many measures taken at the local level produce major health benefits. Where there are public green spaces and forests, people use them to walk, play, and cycle, turning physical activity into an integral part of their daily lives, reducing the risk of injuries and the urban heat-island effect, reducing stress levels and noise pollution, and increasing social life. Public green space can also contribute to flood management *(246)*.

The health sector is one of the most intensive users of energy, a major source of employment and a significant producer of waste, including biological and radioactive waste. Important opportunities to improve the environment are therefore emerging from the greening of health services. Hospitals and clinics can achieve substantial health and economic benefits through energy efficiency measures such as developing low-energy medical devices, using renewable energy, conserving water and storing it safely on site, improving the management of procurement, recycling waste and using locally grown food. The health sector also has an essential part to play in mitigating the effects of climate change and in reducing environmental exposure by taking steps to limit its own significant climate footprint and its negative impact on the environment. Nevertheless, the potential and capacity for greening health services varies greatly between countries, with a west–east gradient. Adopting appropriate legislation, providing incentives to increase the institutional capacity to make initial investments, providing renewable and energy-efficient technology, and raising awareness can all help to overcome the obstacles to implementation.

The evidence on how green development can benefit health and equity is increasing, as the topic attains a higher profile *(251)*. Important areas of research include the health effects of new technologies and innovation, and the health and equity benefits of green and inclusive growth policies in other sectors. Green growth and prosperity will not necessarily be inclusive or catalyse poverty reduction, unless they are accompanied by approaches to benefit poor people and to focus on health as an integral part of a green development approach. Economic affordability is but one component of inclusive growth and equitable access. Several economic support measures have been proposed, across a variety of sectors, to deal with access to water, food, sanitation and household energy. These range from direct financial support and technological improvements to ensuring minimum service provision for the people most in need.

Demonstrating the relationship between sustainable development and health is a powerful argument to support climate change mitigation and adaptation in particular, and sustainable development in general. Health outcomes can be measured and can generate public and political interest. Health will be a critical component in how the progress and impact of sustainable development are tracked after Rio+20.

Expanding interdisciplinary and intersectoral collaboration between human, environmental and animal health will enhance the efficacy of public health. This requires working to fully implement multilateral environmental agreements, as well as the recommendations of the European environment and health process; expeditiously expanding the scientific knowledge base; assessing the effects on health of policies in various sectors, especially those affecting both health and the environment; ensuring the continual development and adaptation of services for environment and health; and encouraging the health sector to act in an environmentally more responsible manner.

The urban environment

Models of health care vary across the Region. In broad terms, central and regional governments usually directly administer hospital treatment and care; primary care is usually decentralized. Local governments often take primary responsibility for managing long-term illness and disability, administering or directly providing many housing, health and social support services, especially for older people. Public health and environment and health functions were previously often combined at the municipal level, but these functions are currently more likely to be separated, although in some countries they are being reunited.

About 69% of the people in the European Region live in urban settings. Living and working in urban areas affects health and health prospects both positively and negatively, through a complex array of types of exposure and mechanisms. In addition, cities concentrate population groups with various demographic, economic and social characteristics, some with particular health risks and vulnerability.

Urban areas provide great opportunities for individuals and families to prosper and can promote health through enhanced access to services, culture and recreation. Nevertheless, although cities are the engines of economic prosperity and often the location of the greatest wealth in the country, they can also concentrate poverty and ill health *(265)*. Urban health has emerged in recent years as a framing paradigm for a field of research and policy that serves to unite and focus the variety of forces determining the health of city-dwellers *(266)*.

City living can affect health through the physical and built environment, the social environment and access to services and support. The quality of housing, neighbourhood design, the density of development and mix of land uses, access to green space and facilities, recreational areas, cycling lanes, air quality, noise and exposure to toxic substances have all been shown to affect the health and well-being of the population in many different ways. Some circumstances of urban life, especially segregation and poverty, contribute to and reinforce these discrepancies, by imposing disproportionate exposure to health-adverse and socially undesirable patterns of response to economic and social deprivation. The numbers of older people living in cities is increasing, which requires rethinking urban planning and standards for providing services *(267)*.

Most local governments in the European Region have a general duty to promote the well-being of their citizens and provide equal and similar access to municipal resources and opportunities. Cities can achieve this through their influence in several domains, such as health, social services, the environment, education, the economy, housing, security, transport and sport. Intersectoral partnerships and community empowerment initiatives can be implemented more easily at the local level with the active support of local governments. The Healthy Cities network provides many examples of good practice.

Cities significantly influence people's health and well-being through various policies and interventions, including those addressing social exclusion and support; healthy and active living (such as cycle lanes and smoke-free public areas); safety and environmental issues for children and older people; working conditions; preparedness to deal with the consequences of climate change; exposure to hazards and nuisances; healthy urban planning and design (neighbourhood planning, removal of architectural barriers, accessibility and proximity of services); and participatory and inclusive processes for citizens (268).

Applying the "urban lens" has several implications for those who are concerned with action for health and well-being:

- understanding and taking into account the urban specificity and distribution of the socioeconomic and environmental determinants of health;
- addressing the conditions that increase people's potential exposure and vulnerability to communicable and noncommunicable diseases;
- addressing the changing demographic and social landscape of cities, such as the ageing of the population and migration;
- incorporating urban health issues in national health policies, strategies and plans; and
- acknowledging the importance of the role of local governments in promoting health and health equity in all local policies and whole-of-society engagement.

Local leadership for health and well-being and the role of mayors and civic leaders

For numerous reasons, local governments are uniquely placed to provide leadership for health and well-being. Many of the social determinants of health operate at the local and community level. For this reason, in the complex world of multiple tiers of government, with numerous public and private stakeholders, local governments do have the capacity to influence the determinants of health and inequalities. They are well positioned to influence land use, building standards and water and sanitation systems, and to enact and enforce restrictions on tobacco use and occupational health and safety regulations. Second, many local governments have the capability to develop and implement integrated strategies for health promotion. Third, their democratic mandate conveys authority and sanctions their power to convene partnerships and encourage contributions from many sectors. Fourth, local governments have daily contact with citizens and are closest to their concerns and priorities. They present unique opportunities for partnering with the private and not-for-profit sectors, civic society and citizens' groups. Fifth, local governments have the capacity to mobilize local resources and to deploy them to create more opportunities for poor and vulnerable population groups and to protect and promote the rights of all urban residents.

Nevertheless, leadership is not limited to understanding how one's authority and potential areas of influence can promote health and reduce health inequities. Local leadership for health means having a vision and an understanding of the importance of health in social and economic development; having the commitment and conviction to forge new partnerships and alliances; promoting accountability for health by statutory and non-statutory local actors, aligning local action with national policies; anticipating and planning for change; and ultimately acting as a guardian, facilitator, catalyst, advocate and defender of the right to the highest level of health for all residents *(249,269)*.

Effective leadership for health and well-being requires political commitment, a vision and strategic approach, supportive institutional arrangements, and networking and connecting with others who are working towards similar goals *(270,271)*. The true power of local leaders to promote health and well-being does not lie within their formal powers. Rather, it comes from their ability to inspire and to lead. By harnessing the combined efforts of a multitude of actors, local governments can multiply their power and make a true difference to the health and well-being of local communities. These essential elements of effective action are aimed at changing how individuals, communities, nongovernmental organizations, the private sector and local governments understand and make decisions about health and health equity.

The social environment: social determinants of and assets for health

Building resilience is a key factor in protecting and promoting health at both the individual and community levels. The health of any individual is closely linked to the health of the larger community. Communities play a vital role in providing health promotion and disease prevention activities and ensuring the social inclusion of people with chronic diseases and people with disabilities. This role is influenced and shaped by the complex inter-relationship between natural, built and social environments. Policy action to make such environments healthier will help communities, and the people in them, to be empowered in their choices and to sustain their own health.

Given these rapidly changing environments, focusing on continually striving to improve living and working conditions is key to supporting health. At the macro level, social and economic policies need to create environments which ensure that people at all times of life are better able to reach their full health potential. At the micro level, action initiated in specific settings where people live, love, work and play – homes, schools, workplaces, leisure environments, care services and older people's homes – can be very effective. The WHO Healthy Cities and Communities movement provides extensive examples of how to build such resilience, especially by involving local people and generating community ownership of health issues. Other settings-based networks – such as health-promoting schools or workplaces – provide similar experiences. Health and social services, and especially primary health care services reaching out to families in their homes, to workers at their workplaces and to local community groups, are important entry points for systematically supporting individuals and communities over the lifespan and especially during critical periods *(235,272)*.

People cannot be empowered by others but can only empower themselves by acquiring more powers, making use of their own inherent assets, facilitated by external structures and life circumstances. Communities can support individuals and patients by establishing social networks and by mobilizing social support, which together promote cohesion between individuals and can support people through difficult transitions in life and periods of vulnerability and illness. Communities should provide structures, resources and opportunities for individuals, groups and neighbourhoods to network, to become better organized and build capacity with other actors, to develop leadership and to take responsibility for their health, their diseases and their lives. In recent years, tools have been developed and on-the-ground experiences have been accumulated in this domain. Several examples have been reported by the literature on health assets and on community resilience *(273,274)*. These innovations aim to identify available assets for individuals and communities to solve local issues in a sustainable way and ensure that external support through welfare and other service can be used more effectively. For example, the recently formed Assets Alliance in Scotland is a platform for sharing assets and guiding the Scottish government and national agencies on policy development *(275)*.

The existence of an adequate social protection system influences health and health equity. Government social spending substantially affects poverty rates which, in turn, are associated with higher mortality, especially among women and children, and particularly women with a low educational level. Social protection influences health among adults, especially in low- and medium-income countries.

Whole-of-government responsibility for health requires that the effects on health be fundamentally considered in developing all regulatory policies *(47)*. The persistent and often increasing socially determined inequity in health requires integrated action and a systems approach *(276,277)*. Strong political commitment, effective and high-performing health systems and coherence across government policies are all needed, as are well-functioning institutions capable of influencing policy-making across health and other policy sectors. Systematically targeting public policies and private initiatives, and aligning the financial, human and environmental resources, will mobilize action for better health and well-being and its equal distribution in society *(49,51,278)*.

A key aim of policy should be to maintain the minimum standards needed for healthy living. Evidence shows that social spending is more generous in countries with more universal social protection policies and higher rates of labour force participation. Specific actions to be recommended on social protection include ensuring that women and children have access to the minimum income needed for healthy living; that social spending is sufficiently generous, especially among women with a low educational level; that social protection systems in low- and medium-income countries are generous and universal; and that active labour market programmes, linked to generous social protection, promote high rates of labour force participation.

Addressing the social determinants of health and tackling health inequities require going further than the traditional model for providing health and social care. In addition to providing public services to address the deficiencies in a given community, efforts should also be directed towards harnessing any inherent assets and support that may exist within communities and which can enhance and complement the offerings of the public sector *(27)*. Many well-meant programmes to promote health and reduce socially caused inequity in health fail because they are not based on such a system-wide approach.

As health assets relate to the social determinants of health, asset-based approaches have the potential to overcome some of the existing barriers to maximizing health and well-being and reducing health inequities. Such approaches are strongly linked to health promotion and intervention models and emphasize the importance of strengthening protective and promoting factors for individual and community health by identifying the skills, strengths, capacities and knowledge of individuals and the social capital of communities. These models focus on identifying what assets are available to protect, maintain and promote the health of individuals and communities. The aim is to maximize these assets in order to solve local health issues in a sustainable way and ensure that any external support (such as providing services to enhance health and well-being) can be used more effectively *(279–281)*.

Efforts to reduce vulnerability and counter the operation of exclusionary processes are important. Smarter governance is necessary to enable communities to steer governments and other agencies to pursue health and well-being as collective goals. New structures for governance and leadership are needed to do this. Rather than building capacity from the outside, empowering social, political and economic systems should be created that release capacity within organizations, professional groups, communities, families and disadvantaged groups. Creating this empowerment requires various types of knowledge and evidence, built on the experience and interpretation of people in the groups and communities affected.

These approaches help to translate such concepts and principles into local action. The goal is public investment in local communities, building on local strengths and assets to raise levels of aspiration, build resilience and release potential *(282)*. Thus, asset-based approaches are an integral part of health promotion and should become an integral part of strategies to improve health and reduce health inequities *(283,284)*.

Raising awareness in communities, families and individuals that there are opportunities for change and support, and that everybody can help to remove barriers to a better and healthier life, can offer greater freedom for people with health problems, in particular for individuals with chronic diseases and those with disabilities, and foster their meaningful contribution to the community. The aim is to recognize and enhance the roles of different stakeholders and enhance follow-up and accountability. Actions include: involving patient and family caregiver associations and related nongovernmental organizations in providing care for patients and supporting them with public funds; building supportive communities to enable people to live as independently as possible; promoting support for disease self-management at workplaces; strengthening means of social support in communities that encourage participation and contact with people with chronic diseases and with disabilities; and initiating and funding anti-stigma programmes, to change negative attitudes towards people with chronic conditions and people with disabilities. Health literacy is a promising actionable concept that addresses the dynamic interaction between individuals and the environments in which they live and work, focusing on learning and skill development for health, including the ability to navigate the complex social and health systems to benefit one's health. Health literacy applies a life-course approach, is sensitive to cultural and contextual factors and is concerned with both individuals and organizations.

Informal caregivers provide the largest share of care. Supporting their role, training them and protecting their well-being create positive outcomes for the health both of caregivers and of the people for whom they care. Key action points are to provide official recognition, financial support and social security benefits to informal caregivers; to involve informal caregivers in decision-making processes on health policy and services; to provide home visits and regular communication between professionals and informal caregivers, including assessment of health and safety conditions and technical aids; to use informal caregivers' experience of the individual being cared for when training professional caregivers; and to provide mental health protection measures for informal caregivers, such as opportunities for flexible and part-time work, peer support and self-help, and training and tools to evaluate caregivers' own mental health needs.

Part 3

Health 2020: enhancing effective implementation – requirements, pathways and continuous learning

Introduction

Part 3 describes the requirements and pathways that can support effective implementation of Health 2020. Two challenges go hand in hand – governance of the health system and health systems strengthening, which together are referred to as health governance; and the joint action of health and non-health sectors, public and private sectors, and citizens for a common purpose – to promote governance for health. Implementing Health 2020 requires movement on several core elements: leadership; strategic intent (expressed through national and subnational health policies); working together through partnerships; developing whole-of-society and whole-of-government responsibility for health; monitoring, evaluation and public health research; and a strong role for WHO.

Making it happen – the challenges facing policy-makers

In taking Health 2020 forward, countries will not only face different contexts and starting-points but also need to have the capacity to adapt to both anticipated and unanticipated conditions under which policies must be implemented. The world today is very different from the former Health for All policy environments – this document, as well as the study on governance for health, has already drawn attention to challenges such as global interdependence and connectedness, the quickening pace of change, the added complexity of the policy environment, and the increase in uncertainty. New policy approaches and tools are needed to work effectively in such a world *(285)*.

Member States will choose different approaches and align their actions and choices on their particular political, social, epidemiological and economic realities, their capacity for developing and implementing policy, and their respective histories and cultures. Member States are encouraged to analyse and critically appraise where they stand in relation to the Health 2020 policy framework and whether their policy instruments, legislative, organizational, human resource and fiscal situations and measures support or impede the implementation of Health 2020. This includes an appreciation of system complexity, capacity, performance and dynamics. Health 2020 sets out the present, emerging and future issues that need to be addressed, but it also highlights the fact that policy-makers are challenged to accommodate unforeseen issues as well as changes in context that will have an impact on policy goals. Continuous analysis and policy adjustments will be necessary, as will the readiness to terminate policies that are no longer relevant or effective.

Implementing Health 2020 will be demanding. A recent study undertaken by the WHO Regional Office for Europe to support the development of Health 2020 and facilitate its implementation considered the various public health commitments made by Member States between 1990 and 2010. These amounted to an impressive number of resolutions, policy statements and legally binding instruments. Most Health 2020 topics had been addressed, although some appeared to have needed more attention, such as older people, the management of selected noncommunicable diseases, and the economic implications of health and disease. The authors questioned the sustainability of such an approach, identified the challenges of monitoring and evaluating implementation, and raised the possibilities of repetition and duplication.

In such a complex environment, seven approaches have been suggested to support policy-making.

- *Integrated and forward-looking analysis.* If the key factors that affect policy performance are identified and scenarios are drawn up for how these factors might evolve in the future, policies can then be made robust in response to a range of anticipated conditions, and indicators can be developed to help trigger important policy adjustments when needed.
- *Multistakeholder deliberation.* This entails a collective and collaborative public effort to examine an issue from different viewpoints before making a decision. Deliberative processes strengthen policy design by fostering acknowledgement of common values, shared commitment and emerging issues and by providing a comprehensive understanding of causal relationships.
- *Automatic policy adjustment.* Some of the inherent variability in socioeconomic and ecological conditions can be anticipated, and monitoring of key indicators can help trigger important policy adjustments to keep the policy functioning well.
- *Enabling self-organization and social networking.* Ensuring that policies do not undermine existing social capital, creating forums that enable social networking, facilitating the sharing of good practices and removing barriers to self-organization all strengthen the ability of stakeholders to respond to unanticipated events in a variety of innovative ways.
- *Decentralization of decision-making.* Decentralizing the authority and responsibility for decision-making to the lowest effective and accountable unit of governance, whether existing or newly created, can increase the capacity of a policy to perform successfully when confronting unforeseen events.
- *Promoting variation.* Given the complexity of most policy settings, implementing a variety of policies to address the same issue increases the likelihood of achieving the desired outcomes. The diversity of responses also constitutes a common risk management approach, facilitating the ability to perform efficiently in the face of unanticipated conditions.
- *Formal policy review and continuous learning.* Regular review, even when the policy is performing well, and the use of well-designed pilot schemes throughout the life of the policy to test assumptions related to performance, can help to address emerging issues and trigger important policy adjustments.

Leadership, including strengthening the roles of health ministers and the health sector

Leadership for health and health equity is now more important than ever. There are many forms of health leadership, involving many actors: for example, international organizations setting standards and "goalposts"; heads of governments giving priority to health and well-being; health ministers reaching out beyond their sector to ministers in other sectors; parliamentarians expressing an interest in health; business leaders seeking to reorient their business models to take health and well-being into account; civil society organizations drawing attention to shortcomings in disease prevention or in service delivery; academic institutions providing evidence on which health interventions work (and which do not) and research findings for innovation; and local authorities taking on the challenge of health in all policies. Individuals such as philanthropists or media personalities have also increasingly taken on leadership roles for health and equity issues and have campaigned with great effect.

Such leadership for health in the 21st century requires new skills, often using influence, rather than direct control, to achieve results. Much of the authority of health leaders in the future will reside not only in their position in the health system but also in their ability to convince others that health and well-being are highly relevant in all sectors. Leadership will be not only individual but also institutional, collective, community-centred and collaborative. Such forms of leadership are already in evidence. Groups of stakeholders are coming together to address key health challenges at the global, regional, national and local levels, such as the global movement on HIV. Similar movements are emerging around noncommunicable diseases, environmental health and health promotion.

Health ministers and ministries have a vital role to play here. Their strong leadership is key for all the actions necessary to advance health, including: developing and implementing national and subnational health strategies focused on improving health and well-being; advocating for and achieving effective intersectoral working for health; engaging the active participation of all stakeholders; delivering high-quality and effective core public health functions and health care services; and defining and monitoring standards of performance within a framework of transparent accountability.

Their responsibility for effective, responsive and efficient health services also contributes substantially to equitable improvement in health. Health services themselves contribute to health and well-being outcomes, and this contribution can be expected to grow over time as the technological capacity of health services increases across the whole spectrum of illness and disease. In addition, health services themselves are a powerful social determinant of health, in terms of socially distributed inequalities in access and usage.

Developing, implementing and evaluating national and subnational health policies, strategies and plans, drawing on the contribution of various sectors

Health policies focus on the pursuit of specific and measurable health gain, especially the increase of healthy life-years and the ability to live independently with chronic disease. Concern about health is a key policy priority at all levels of governance, requiring an effective and integrated health system serving public health needs and focusing on primary health care. Achieving these goals involves preparing a comprehensive plan for developing health and well-being, including developing and strengthening health services. Related to this is the aim of strengthening intersectoral approaches.

Such planning instruments must transcend delivering only health care and address the broad agenda of improving health and the social determinants of health, as well as the interaction between the health sector and the other sectors of society. A national health strategy – which can take many different forms – can provide an inspirational overarching or "umbrella" policy, involving a comprehensive range of stakeholders and sectors and focusing on improving population health. Such a strategy can support shared values, foster synergy and promote transparency and accountability. For low- and medium-income countries, the process of developing health policies, strategies and plans can also assist donors in health planning work and contribute to effective donor coordination. The process should be informed by a comprehensive health needs assessment that is sensitive to age, gender, social position and condition.

Research and other intelligence shows that many policies and services, despite having an established evidence base (such as reducing salt and saturated fat in diets, increasing taxes on tobacco, detecting and managing hypertension, managing stroke by multidisciplinary teams, and actively managing the third stage of labour), do not reach populations in need. There are many reasons for a failure to apply evidence to policy and practice. Some are technical and arise from the type and nature of the evidence collected; some are organizational and occur when partnerships or cross-sector working is weak; others are political and arise because what the evidence says is not welcomed by those charged with setting priorities and making investment decisions. Response to interventions also depends upon individuals being empowered to sustain the potential benefits.

Of course, evidence is rarely the only or even the principal factor governing how decisions are made. Values and other influences are also important. Nevertheless, there remains scope to scale up the delivery of core cost-effective services and free up resources, but this means efforts must be made to expand evidence-informed interventions aimed at those with greater needs and reduce the delivery of inappropriate care or public health interventions of limited utility. For such an approach to succeed, researchers, policy-makers and practitioners need to work in new and different ways, centred on the co-production of knowledge and evidence that truly meets their respective needs.

In addition to necessary, and often new, funds, a commitment to address the inefficient use of resources in the health sector is vital to secure popular and political support for more spending. Efficiency gains need to be a central part of health plans and strategies rather than a short-term response to budget cuts, because the transition to a new, lower-cost delivery system needs to be carefully managed and may require investment in the short term. The goal is to achieve sustainable efficiency gains, such as improving energy efficiency, shifting more care to outpatient settings, allocating more resources to primary health care and cost-effective public health programmes, cutting the least cost-effective services, and improving the rational use of medicines.

The performance of often fragmented health systems may be mismatched with the rising expectations of societies and citizens. People expect greater participation, empowerment, fairness and respect for human rights in health system delivery. The expectation is for increased domestic expenditure on health, but resources are always limited. Strengthening health systems and health system governance are crucial for meeting these expectations. Health ministers and health ministries, and other national authorities, need help and support in improving health system performance and in increasing accountability and transparency.

Health policy is usually developed through diverse approaches and levels and with differing aims. Mechanistic approaches are not sufficient and in any case have been found wanting. More flexible and integrative approaches are required, which are able to respond rapidly to changing circumstances and to sound evidence of what works well and not so well. Comprehensive development of health strategy is inherently a highly political process, and this has to be acknowledged at every stage.

Political and legal commitments are of crucial importance for ensuring long-term sustainability. Flexibility is needed to adapt to unexpected developments in the political, economic and health environment. The value largely lies in the process. Such strategies are more likely to be implemented if they are made and "owned" by the people who will implement them and if they are aligned with capacity, resources and constraints. The instruments must chart realistic ways of developing capacity and resources by mobilizing partners and stakeholders, who may have competing interests.

Adding value through partnerships and partners for health

Health 2020 will be achieved by combining individual and collective efforts. Key to the success of Health 2020 will be Member States and WHO working closely together and reaching out to engage other partners. The whole-of-government and whole-of-society approaches to improving health and well-being, which are at the core of Health 2020, are grounded in strategies that enhance joined-up government, improve coordination, integration and diffusion of responsibility for health throughout government and society, and aim to empower people at local and community levels. Today's complex health challenges need to be addressed through a multi-level, whole-of-society and whole-of-government approach that, in addition to state and public sector actors, includes civil society, the private sector and the mass media. Success will require a common purpose and broad collaborative efforts by actors across society in every country: governments, nongovernmental organizations, civil society, the private sector, science and academia, health professionals, communities – and every individual.

Today's leaders for health must advocate for and build partnerships for health. These partnerships are a core concept within Health 2020, which adopts a whole-system perspective. Effective partnerships with institutions, citizens and communities, civil society and public and private stakeholders will be essential at several levels, in order to gain insight into local determinants of health, win support for action across all of society and contribute to community development. This is partly about making whole-of-government and intersectoral governance for health work better, and partly about developing broad international, national and local constituencies for health.

Partnerships within and outside government depend on mutual interests and personal relations, as well as on a positive environment in which to operate. There are many types of partnerships built on varied forms of relationship; for example, partnerships may be formal, informal, or mostly technical in nature. The evidence shows how crucially important are the strength, quality and transparency of the links between partners, mechanisms for attributing responsibility and accountability, and, most particularly, arrangements for budget-setting and reporting. These characteristics of partnerships fundamentally affect outcomes and performance.

Across all levels of structures, important issues related to power asymmetries need to be considered. Although many organizations endorse partnerships and acknowledge constituents' interests as being important, research and other analyses demonstrate beyond doubt that not all parties fully embrace partnership, understand each other's cultures, or adhere to the principles they espouse or operational and management principles of good practice. Many of the challenges relate to the need for mechanisms or arrangements to deal with hidden agendas and potential conflicts of interest, and to negotiate the basis of partnerships. Partnership is key in intersectoral governance, but how partners contribute to the information and resource base for decisions may in practice be more hierarchical than horizontal.

Supporting civil society strengthens advocacy for health and equity. The principles and value of building community engagement and empowerment are well recognized, and supporting a diverse civil society of people who often volunteer time and effort freely to contribute to important interventions and approaches is of key importance. Civil society also adds value in being able to communicate with people in unconventional ways. Although governments and official bodies have important roles to play in communicating accurate and credible information, how messages are received from government and civil society can be very different. Civil society can often address complex, sensitive or stigmatized issues in a way that official bodies and authorities cannot, particularly by strengthening engagement with marginalized groups, who may have been poorly reached previously, and by harnessing business sector engagement in an appropriate and ethical manner. Voluntary organizations and self-help groups can also contribute important perspectives and offer practical assistance to those in need. There is a new and expanding role for the social media in articulating and communicating health messages and perceptions.

Partnerships with international organizations active in the European Region are critical in supporting the aims of Health 2020. The role of WHO and its interrelationship with these organizations will rest not only on its pursuit of technical excellence, evidence-informed practice and results-based management but also on its commitment to work with others in helping Member States realize their full health potential. The existing close cooperation between WHO and international organizations is being strengthened still further. These include bodies such as specialized agencies of the United Nations system, the World Bank and regional development banks, OECD, the EU, the Council of Europe, the Global Fund to Fight AIDS, Tuberculosis and Malaria, development agencies and funds, and major nongovernmental organizations. UNICEF is a particular partner in many vital areas of public health, such as maternal and child health, immunization, measures to reinforce health promotion and disease prevention by strengthening health systems and closer monitoring of the health divide.

Working with the EU will provide a strong foundation, great opportunities and additional benefits. The European Commission has published a white paper that proposes fundamental principles and strategic objectives for its action on health *(22)*. This is linked to Article 168 of the Treaty on the Functioning of the European Union, as amended by the Lisbon Treaty *(112)*, which requires that "a high level of human health protection shall be ensured in the definition and implementation of all Union policies and activities".

In addition, EU candidate and potential candidate countries, as well as European Neighbourhood and Partnership Instrument countries, are working to progressively align their legislation and practices with EU policies. This can be very important for implementing Health 2020. The joint declaration by the European Commission and WHO, which includes six "roadmaps" for closer collaboration, is an important step in strengthening their partnership in improving health information, health security and funding for health, as well as in reducing health inequalities, carrying out health research and improving in-country collaboration. Specific initiatives by the European Commission such as the European Innovative Partnership on Active and Healthy Ageing *(286)* will also offer opportunities for collaboration.

Linking with new and evolving types of partnerships for health that are active at various levels of governance across the Region will also provide important support. Substantial contributions are made by innovative cooperation mechanisms, including the Eurasian Economic Community; the South-eastern Europe Health Network and the Northern Dimension; by policy networks such as the WHO European Healthy Cities Network and Regions for Health; by subregional networks within the CIS; and by WHO's health promotion settings networks, including schools, workplaces, hospitals and prisons throughout the Region.

Academic and professional institutions, including medical and other health care professional organizations, WHO collaborating centres and public health networks at regional and country levels, also represent important potential partners.

It is important to look for ways to cooperate appropriately and ethically with the private sector, including the pharmaceutical industry, especially since its involvement is increasing across the European Region. Attitudes towards the private sector vary between and within countries. However, businesses (from the very local to the global) are increasingly involved in every aspect of people's lives. They are in all communities, and at all levels, and their knowledge and understanding of local communities represents an often untapped resource and an asset that, if appropriately harnessed, can contribute significantly to health and well-being. Many small and large businesses are key sponsors of community-level activities, and there is real potential to build further on this. It is clear, however, that their influence can either help to enhance health or undermine it.

The United Nations General Assembly, in Article 44 of its political declaration on the prevention and control of noncommunicable diseases *(180)*, calls on the private sector to strengthen its contribution to preventing and controlling noncommunicable diseases and sets a five-point agenda that includes implementing WHO recommendations to reduce the impact of marketing of foods to children; reformulating food products to provide healthier options (including salt reduction); promoting health in the workforce; and improving access to and affordability of essential medicines and technologies.

Creating and maintaining partnerships for health involves new ways of thinking about organizational form, structure and functioning. Relationships are key and will require open, transparent and respectful dealings between partners. Networked structures may be more appropriate than conventional bureaucratic forms. Methods of decision-making, resource allocation and accountability need to be highly visible and open to scrutiny and influence by everyone.

Creating whole-of-society and whole-of-government responsibility for health work

Capacity for governance for health: by the whole of society and the whole of government, and through health in all policies – applying the governance lens

Whole-of-society and whole-of-government responsibilities for health will be driven by a high degree of political commitment, enlightened public administration and societal support. Making this responsibility meaningful and functional requires concrete intersectoral governance structures that can facilitate the requisite action, with the aim of including, where appropriate, health in all policies, sectors and settings. These intersectoral governance structures are equally relevant for governments, parliaments, administrations, the public, stakeholders and industry.

The aim of a whole-of-society approach is to expand whole-of-government thinking by emphasizing the roles of the private sector and civil society and a wide range of political decision-makers, such as parliamentarians. The policy networks that have emerged within government increasingly extend beyond their boundaries to include other social actors. The whole-of-society approach implies additional capacity for communication and collaboration in complex, networked settings and highlights the role of the media and new forms of communication. Each party must invest resources and competence. By engaging the private sector, civil society, communities and individuals, the whole-of-society approach increases the resilience of communities to withstand threats to their health, security and well-being. As stated by Paquet *(287)*: "Collaboration is the new categorical imperative". The whole-of-society approach goes beyond institutions: it influences and mobilizes local and global culture and mass media, rural and urban communities, and all relevant policy sectors, including education, transport, the environment and even urban design, as can be demonstrated with respect to obesity and the global food system. Whole-of-society approaches are forms of collaborative governance that emphasize coordination through normative values and trust-building among various actors in society. The approaches usually imply steering instruments that are less prescriptive, less committed to a uniform approach, and less centralized and hierarchical. Joint goals and targets, such as *Healthy people 2020* in the United States of America *(288)*, are a good starting point. Many EU policies have a similar basis, given the wide consultation that precedes them, usually involving all relevant stakeholders, public as well as private, although not with the same level of influence.

Nevertheless, governments must retain the ultimate responsibility for and commitment to protecting and promoting the health and well-being of the people they serve and the societies they reflect. At all levels in society, political commitment is absolutely vital to focus the responsibility and accountability for improving health and well-being. Thus, governance for health and health equity will require governments to strengthen the coherence of policies, investment, services and action across sectors and stakeholders. Synergistic policies are required, many of which reside outside health, supported by structures and mechanisms that foster and enable collaboration. Many determinants of health and health equity are shared priorities with other sectors, such as improving educational performance, promoting social inclusion and cohesion, reducing poverty and improving community resilience and well-being. These provide a convening point for action across sectors that will produce benefits for health and health equity *(289)*. There is a clear role for health impact assessment to bring health and other policy outcomes into a common frame of analysis.

Achieving whole-of-government governance for health is difficult and challenging. Much more is required than a simple mandate *(290)*. In addition, the evidence to support intersectoral governance is often scarce, partial, inconclusive or anecdotal. However, progress is possible, as shown by lessons from the fields of sustainability and development. A key action area is developing new or strengthened instruments and mechanisms that ensure equity of voice and perspectives in decision-making processes. Effective governance for health employs collaborative models of working to increase resource flows; to improve the distribution of determinants, affecting the opportunity to be healthy; to redress the current patterns and magnitude of health inequities; and to reduce the risks and effects of disease and premature mortality across the whole population.

The findings of the Task Group on Governance and Delivery Mechanisms (291), one of the task groups linked to the European review of social determinants of health and the health divide *(17)*, indicate that interventions to address the social determinants of health and tackle health inequities usually require improved systems of governance and delivery. These will need to operate at all levels of governance, involving both the whole of society and the whole of government, and to provide both a national as well as a local context for action on health. The Task Group has identified several main reasons why governance and delivery systems fail to address the social determinants of health and related health inequities:

- a failure to conceptualize and act on the full causal pathway leading to the desired outcome of reduced health inequities (conceptual failure);
- a failure to construct an effective delivery chain and supportive incentives and organizational mechanisms capable of delivering improved outcomes in terms of social determinants of health and health inequities (delivery chain failure); and
- a failure to develop a control strategy that oversees the overall delivery process (government control strategy failure).

This last failure is often linked to weak capacity to identify and quickly rectify a wide range of shortcomings, such as organizational, financial and legislative inadequacies and other causes of underperformance.

Thus, Member States may consider several preconditions and measures needed to "make it happen" and increase their governance performance. A review of studies that have analysed progress in this domain throws light on important lessons and opportunities to reduce the failures outlined above *(291)*. In making progress towards adopting a whole-of-society and whole-of-government approach to taking action for reducing health inequities, several innovative practices and tools are now available for countries to consider and adapt to their specific contexts, nationally and subnationally.

The following principal developments may be especially relevant.

- *Government structures*. At the cabinet table, ministers can develop joint policies either under the auspices of the head of government or through collaboration between selected ministries. Cabinet subcommittees may be formed to deal with health issues as part of a whole-of-government approach, with mechanisms to promote a common understanding of solutions. Institutional platforms can be used, such as a jointly staffed health policy unit embedded in the prime minister's office, or joint committees or working groups. Interdepartmental committees may facilitate the provision of evidence and the development and coordination of policy. Keeping the issues of health and development alive and influential may require a small, dedicated resource unit moving freely across communities and sectors, creating and promoting regular dialogue and platforms for debate. Providing a legal mandate reflects high-level support for action on the social determinants of health.
- *Mega-ministries and ministerial mergers*. These have been introduced in an attempt to enhance the efficiency and coherence of political and administrative work in government. While the argument for such changes might appear compelling, the evidence for increased intersectoral coherence is not.
- *Public health ministers*. These may have an explicit intersectoral mandate to support whole-of-government action for health. They may be supported by a high-level national steering committee composed of representatives of key national, regional and local authorities and agencies.
- *Ministerial links and strategic alliances*. These bring together otherwise separated if not isolated policy fields at top decision-making level. There are different approaches to establishing policy coherence at the cabinet level. Such cross-government alliances among policy sectors can be incentivized through a range of mechanisms that are mutually reinforcing and hold key sectors accountable. One approach sees cabinet ministers together developing a policy, with each of them owning a limited number

of targets in the joint policy, aligning sub-targets with each other so that policy goals do not conflict. Another possibility for establishing ministerial links is to commission policy frameworks from the finance ministry for each ministry. Such mechanisms for ensuring joint targets and common shared goals, backed up by statements of mutual responsibility, are proving effective in this regard, particularly when they are understood as being one way for organizations to share risks and hold each other accountable *(293)*.

- *Shared and pooled budgets*. The current economic difficulties that governments are facing throughout the European Region may force policy sectors to work in a different and more cooperative manner, thus making the notions of "whole-of-government" and "whole-of-society" operational and able to address issues related to health inequities and their social determinants. Countries are already using some new mechanisms that can help build and sustain strategic alliances across sectors. Shared and pooled budgets among policy sectors can promote the development of new accounting methods and the creation of new funds. Examples are found in South Australia and are also emerging in Europe, mainly at the subnational level *(294)*. These mechanisms can integrate financial incentives and reward systems that foster the vertical and horizontal integration needed to reduce health inequities. In some cases, they can also include sharing and rotating human and other resources across sectoral boundaries, as a means of strengthening intersectoral collaboration and trust *(295)*.
- *Joint review of policies and interventions*. These tools are increasingly used in whole-of-government approaches, in order to promote intersectoral action and cooperation. For example, some countries in the Region involved in action plans to improve the health of the Roma population use joint reviews of policies, and they have been recommended notably in the four key policy areas of education, housing, employment and health *(296)*.
- *Evidence support*. Evidence support helps people develop a common understanding of facts, figures, analysis and interpretations. This creates common ground for dialogue and evaluation of joined-up policies, programmes and projects, to allow shared learning and mutual adjustment as these policies are developed and implemented and to sustain commitment and sustainability over time *(291)*.
- *Reaching out*. Governments need to reach out when trying to engage people, patients and societal stakeholders, including the private sector as appropriate. Public consultations, state health conferences and thematic platforms have served this purpose. Such advocacy can relate to government policies, laws and regulations that are designed to favourably modify health-related issues such as taxation, marketing and advertising arrangements. Advocacy may aim not only to induce acceptance of legal changes but also to promote a shift in attitudes, culture, and social and physical environments

Policy implications for the successful use of intersectoral governance structures

The literature and cases on which research is based provide insights into the non-mechanistic nature of intersectoral governance structures. They are not tools that can be used regardless of the context or circumstances prevailing at any particular time. Their successful use and achievement of the desired results depend on a variety of factors.

- *Political will*. Given the need for ministerial instigation or attendance, mechanisms such as ministerial links, cabinet committees and parliamentary committees all inherently require political will. These governance structures cannot exist without a high level of political engagement and commitment. For bureaucratic structures, such as interdepartmental committees and units, political will is not an essential requirement; however, the presence of political support or interest (such as the request for regular ministerial briefings) enhances their ability to remain active and relevant.

- *Political importance of the specific health issues identified.* This is a key consideration for selecting a governance mechanism, especially one that requires political will. The evidence for this comes from cabinet and parliamentary committees, since they are primarily set up in response to politically important issues, where widespread support for action is necessary.
- *Immediacy of the problem.* Both joint budgeting and the engagement of industry are good options for tackling immediate problems. Although long-term sustainability is a challenge for joint budgeting, these options are frequently used for short-term projects. Industry links are usually formed around a specific health issue and can therefore develop quickly. Parliamentary committees usually require a time-limited response from government to their findings, which suggests that they provide solutions in the short to medium term. Cabinet committees, however, offer more long-term solutions across different sectors and, depending on the nature of the policy or investment decision, may extend beyond the term of a government.
- *Leadership.* Establishing cabinet committees requires strong leadership from the office of the prime minister or highest government official, to provide both the structure and terms of reference and a supportive rationale for consideration of broad policy options of cross-departmental significance. Similarly, mergers and mega-ministries require good leadership and a strong minister to manage change. Mergers that are designed to implement an identifiable policy strategy, supported by an identifiable leadership (body or person), are more likely to be effective. Leadership is considered to be the single most important ingredient for stakeholder engagement, especially when it comes to successfully managing tensions and mediating conflicts in the network, in order to allow the dialogue and collaboration between competing interests to continue. Careful consideration needs to be given to possible power imbalances between stakeholders, so as to determine who is more appropriate to lead the engagement process. Power and resource imbalances have the potential to derail stakeholder engagement. Finally, clear and managed governance structures with defined roles and responsibilities are imperative for effective engagement with industry.
- *Context.* The broader context in which the governance structure is being implemented should be considered. The examples of contextual conditions that were raised in the case studies *(291)* reflect the potential for aligning interests. Context in this case not only refers to the political landscape but is also situational. It includes focusing events, policy images and internal or external shocks at a point in time that create a window of opportunity for effecting intersectoral governance structure and action.
- *Resources.* Resources are a condition for the effectiveness of governance structures. Although resources are certainly linked to some of the other factors, such as the practicalities of implementation, the availability of funds to implement and support the operations of intersectoral governance

structures is an unavoidable aspect when considering their feasibility and capacity to fulfil their objectives. Mergers and mega-ministries are associated with significant costs, and the benefits are uncertain. In essence, reorganizing a system is expensive. Alternatively, joint budgeting may be fostered by demonstrating an economic case for action, in which ministries may be able to provide more detailed information on the costs and benefits related to joint programmes for each participating sector, as a justification and incentive for intersectoral governance.

- *Implementation practicalities*. Many practical issues need to be considered when implementing a governance structure. For example, the activities of interdepartmental committees need to take place in concert with other interdepartmental activities (such as copying other departments into correspondence), in order to reinforce the links between departments. Interdepartmental units need to be a credible ally to at least some interests within the affected sectors. A combination of units and committees within the context of a political mechanism such as a ministerial committee should be a powerful and effective mechanism. Mergers and mega-ministries work better when the merged units are not too organizationally different and when a smaller unit is merged into a larger one and in the process submits to the policy directions of the larger unit. Ensuring the support of an effective group of civil servants within the relevant government departments, including but not limited to an efficient cabinet secretariat, is critical to the optimum functioning of a standing cabinet committee, in terms of its ability to facilitate dialogue on identified matters of cross-departmental importance.

Capacity for tackling the social determinants of health and the health divide – applying the equity lens

Inequities in health cannot be reduced without addressing inequities in the causes of ill health: social divisions, unequal exposure to harm and differential levels of resilience. New systems of governance and delivery are also required, operating at all levels of governance. Countries may use approaches aimed at achieving health equity in all policies as a key to informing further action to address the social determinants of health and reduce health inequalities.

Delivering improved and equitable health outcomes means that multiple levels, systems and sectors must collaborate to address the social determinants of health and reduce health inequities. Numerous governance structures are needed in parallel. Part 2 of *Health 2020* has described the importance of governing through collaboration and through a mix of regulation, persuasion and citizen engagement, and modernizing and strengthening public health systems. The Task Group on Governance and Delivery Mechanisms *(291)* makes several specific recommendations to increase countries' capacity to implement actions that address the social determinants of health and apply the health equity lens in policy-making.

Among these recommendations, the following seem especially important, regardless of the structure of health systems and the levels of centralization or decentralization of policy-making in a country. The key requirements for implementation include the country's capacity to take action that addresses the social determinants of health and the health divide. Several general requirements need to be met *(296)*:

- the availability of relevant data on the magnitude and trends of health inequities in the country, their variations nationally and subnationally, and their main determinants;

- the existence or development of explicit equity-oriented objectives and targets that are directly linked to the policies, action and financial resources needed for implementation;
- a realistic assessment of possibilities and constraints, with special attention paid to external unhealthy policies that may generate or exacerbate inequities in health;
- an adequate management capacity for implementation, including efficient and effective mechanisms for applying health equity in all policies, intersectoral collaboration, and coordination and consistency of action at national and subnational levels; and
- the development of appropriate accountability mechanisms: for example, parliamentary committees can be an important advocate for intersectoral governance for health.

Delivery systems for measures to tackle health inequities must include characteristics that demonstrate evidence of:

- a defined "delivery chain" for agreed interventions;
- clear ownership and active cross-sectoral management of programmes;
- appropriate levers and incentives for both health and non-health systems to deliver reductions in health inequalities;
- a performance management system with clear metrics that is capable of giving strong leadership and direction to all sectors;
- research and evaluation of programme outcomes;
- sustainable financing and professional and citizen training;
- political support and statutory responsibilities for new civic roles in owning and managing the delivery of effective programmes;
- high public visibility and citizen engagement by the state and other sectors;
- annual reporting, development support and public scrutiny of health inequalities; and
- outcomes at all levels of governance, but particularly at those of counties and municipalities.

Health equity in all policies seeks to ensure that government decision-making processes take account of and are accountable for the distributional impact of such decisions on the health of the population. Accountability mechanisms designed to ensure health equity in all policies need to be in place. In this sense, accountability means ensuring that arrangements are in place for stakeholders and regulators to hold to account those to whom responsibilities have been given. Frameworks for holding to account those responsible for action on the social determinants of health should be aligned with recommendations for reducing health inequities *(293)*.

It is recognized that countries are at very different points in terms of health, health equity and socioeconomic development. Yet clear strategies are required to redress the current patterns and magnitude of health inequities by taking action on the social determinants of health. While this may limit what is feasible in the short term and the timescale for addressing specific issues, it should not affect the long-term aspirations of the strategy.

Unfortunately, accountability mechanisms to monitor and act on trends in health inequities remain underdeveloped in Europe. According to the findings of a report on governance for health equity and the social determinants of health *(289)*, hard instruments such as laws and regulations combined with softer mechanisms, including joint reviews, offer the most promise for sustaining the intersectoral implementation of policies to address the social determinants of health. The report highlights several promising practices related to accountability for health equity. Norway's 2011 Public Health Act is a good example of using laws to incentivize other sectors to consider the health and equity effects of their actions and to take them into account when planning, delivering and reviewing policies and services at both national and local levels. However, such mechanisms are often most effective when backed up by other instruments that hold other sectors to account and incentivize joint action. The nature and mix of measures used to hold sectors to account for their effects on health and the determinants of health equity depend on the prevailing governance norms and systems.

Support to evaluate and strengthen overall governance capacity to address the social determinants of health and the health divide

Most countries state that equity and fairness are core values guiding decision-making, but often insufficient attention is explicitly paid to the health and equity impact of public policies and the processes and mechanisms that underpin policy and investment decisions. The coherence of action across sectors and stakeholders needs to be strengthened, in order to increase the resources available to redress the current patterns and magnitude of health inequities. This will improve the distribution of determinants, achieve greater equity in health and level up the gradient. To support this, collaborative models of working are required that are capable of sustaining these increased resources.

Addressing the social determinants of health and the health divide requires strong political commitment, effective and equity-oriented health systems, strong public health programmes and infrastructure, and coherence across government policies. Countries need well-functioning institutions that are capable of supporting policy-making across health and other sectors. Governance capacity is needed to manage stakeholder inputs from ministries, academia and research, nongovernmental organizations and civil society organizations. Several countries have already requested support to increase their overall capacity in this domain *(297)*. In operational terms, the support is designed *(298)*:

- to analyse the current situation of governance in the country to address the social determinants of health and health inequities;
- to reach agreement on short- and medium-term action to strengthen the current performance of governance;
- to identify and implement specific actions through national or subnational efforts and, if needed, international cooperation to strengthen country capacity; and
- to ensure that these actions are periodically and systematically reviewed.

In all cases, the aim is to capture learning and to strengthen the evidence base for effective policy and governance responses that can sustain action to improve health equity over time. Although the wider social behavioural sciences are increasingly being used to improve specific interventions with various population groups, they are also helping to enhance upstream issues such as tackling the social determinants of health. For example, an increasing focus on behavioural aspects can inform and assist approaches to policy advocacy and formulation, and the related strategic analysis and planning. It is critically important to integrate equity into local government structures, including both urban and rural governance, and to, develop local solutions to tackle long-standing patterns of social inequities in health.

In order to support governance for health, better ways of measuring health and well-being are required, considering both objective and subjective data and applying equity and sustainability lenses when developing policy. Practical ways forward include introducing new methods of measurement, as well as new types of public health reporting using modern technologies, to promote political, professional and public debate and accountability. Another need is for the systematic collection of robust evidence about how a multitude of policies affect health and how health affects other policies.

The development of equity-oriented targets at national level should be undertaken as part of a political process involving all relevant stakeholders. However, this in turn requires the development of a monitoring framework, with indicators that are based on data that are fit for purpose. This includes monitoring the social distribution of exposures (risk factors), outcomes and health system responses, as well as the impact of population-based interventions.

New demands for technical assistance from countries and the WHO response

Countries use different entry points to tackle health inequities and their social determinants. This depends on their level of development, structure of health policy-making, level of centralization or decentralization of management of health systems, including public health infrastructure and interventions, and other country-context factors. Nevertheless, countries' efforts in this domain need to be underpinned by a social determinants approach. Requests for technical assistance from WHO to increase country capacity to address the social determinants of health and related health inequities have increased continually in the past decade *(299)*. These requests are likely to increase further with the adoption of Health 2020. The WHO Regional Office for Europe will therefore need to meet increased and diversified demands for technical support.

- *Support to integrate health equity objectives into country development strategies.* Some Member States are already requesting technical support to integrate health equity objectives into their existing or planned social and economic policies and programmes for economic development *(277)*.
- *Support with using an approach based on the social determinants of health to increase performance in disease-specific programmes.* Countries increasingly realize that many disease-specific programmes need to address not only downstream but also upstream factors to ensure better prevention and performance *(300–302)*.
- *Support for group-specific strategies.* Group-specific approaches include major population groups such as children, older people, marginalized groups and people with a high risk of social exclusion and poor health. Group-specific strategies typically need to be combined with approaches based on social determinants of health.
- *Support for integrated learning approaches and new thinking.* Countries are interested in finding ways to build on and test out learning from across the social behavioural sciences and apply this in practice, especially

harnessing the potential insights from areas such as strategic social marketing, behavioural economics and neuroscience.

- *Support to integrate approaches based on gender equity and human rights into country development strategies and national policies and programmes.* Although health equity objectives need to be integrated with gender and human rights, experience shows that specific capacity-building efforts are needed to address these issues. Member States are requesting mechanisms for ensuring the monitoring of and accountability for human rights, and for gender mainstreaming (such as gender analysis, gender budgeting, gender training and gender impact assessment). The WHO Regional Office for Europe is working on an integrated approach to address these cross-cutting issues.

Capacity-building to improve the performance of policies and governance in addressing the social determinants of health and health inequities

The future capacity-building requested by Member States needs to focus on solving problems and developing expertise to address the complex area of social determinants of health and reduce the health divide within and among countries. This should be based on fostering partnerships between countries and European and international institutions, developing expertise in tackling common problems and improving practice. Such capacity-building efforts would include:

- undertaking structured learning exchanges between countries to address common challenges, cross-fertilize learning and enrich national and local policy;
- using an open-source approach to accelerate capacity in applying governance solutions through multicountry and regional policy dialogues, workshops and online communities of learning; and
- highlighting new and emerging issues that influence performance in the area of addressing the social determinants of health and generating the most promising responses through policy simulation, partnership panels and evidence consortia.

Monitoring, evaluation and priorities for public health research

All policies and actions to improve health need a firm knowledge base, and implementing Health 2020 will require the evidence base for health action to be improved. Policy-makers need trustworthy, up-to-date information on health and well-being status, on health needs and on health system goals and outcomes. Health information is a policy resource that is vital to health planning, implementation and evaluation. Health-related information generated by research is needed on health needs and health system functioning, effectiveness, efficiency and outcomes. Developing and evaluating policy depends fundamentally on aligning and combining both health and health-related information.

Health information systems and services need to be developed significantly across the countries in the Region. These include epidemiological systems to support needs assessment, systems to provide outcome information on care processes, and disease-specific systems such as cancer registries.

The WHO Regional Office for Europe works to assist countries in their assessments and technical improvements and by providing health information to countries through:

- working with international partners, including the EU and OECD, to ensure the standardization, international comparability and quality of health data;
- working with a network of health agencies dealing with health information and evidence; and
- actively compiling, interpreting, disseminating and granting easy access to both health data and research evidence.

The databases of the WHO Regional Office for Europe are the main repository of health statistics in the European Region. This key resource provides authoritative health data on the 53 countries in the Region. This enables comparative analysis of the health situation and trends in the Region and surveillance of disease and monitoring of trends in policy areas, including key determinants of health such as alcohol, tobacco and nutrition. WHO is also working to provide a platform for the monitoring of *Health 2020* targets and indicators. These activities are part of WHO's efforts to establish an integrated health information system for Europe together with the EU, as well as a European health information strategy.

Other organizations interested in health in the Region (such as the EU and OECD) provide similar repositories of health data, partially drawing on the WHO databases.

In addition, good health-related research is one of society's most valuable and important tools for laying the foundations of better strategies to improve health and health care. The European Region can draw on the work of many of the world's leading research institutions, but more anticipatory analysis is required. Which are the most cost-effective strategies to preserve health and ensure a sustainable health system? What effects will new technologies have? What are the best strategies to address the health of very old people? What could the health systems of the future look like? What effects will climate change have? What effects will the new communication technologies for health have? Will there be enough physicians and other health care practitioners? What sort of skills and competencies will they need? Will new types of hospitals be needed? What is the potential of home care and community-based care? In short, what are the best ways to prepare for an uncertain future in health?

Health at the crossroads of challenges for the 21st century

The need for countries to act together becomes even more important in an interdependent world. Today, a complex array of global and regional forces can undermine people's health and its determinants, with variable effects. The economic crisis and resulting social consequences illustrate the global interconnectedness of systems and policies. More people than ever before have the chance to attain better health, but no country acting alone can harness the full potential of innovation and change or resolve the challenges to health and well-being that can prevent their attainment among some countries and social groups.

The future prosperity of the European Region depends on countries' willingness and ability to take up the challenges and seize new opportunities for the health and well-being of the whole population of present and future generations. Health 2020 is designed to be an adaptable and practical policy framework, providing a unique platform for joint learning and sharing of expertise and experience between countries. Every country is unique and will pursue these common goals through different means and pathways. Nevertheless, Health

2020 provides a platform for bringing together these different approaches that are united in their core purpose, supported by the reviewing regional targets that have been set collectively. Political commitment to this process is therefore absolutely essential.

New types of partnerships for health are emerging at different levels of governance in the European Region. The principles of governance for health are relevant at the global, regional, national, subnational and local levels. Such networks as the WHO European Healthy Cities Network and the Regions for Health Network, as well as WHO health promotion settings networks including schools, workplaces, hospitals and prisons, are at work throughout the Region.

Health 2020 will be achieved by combining individual and collective efforts. Success requires a common purpose and broad consultative efforts by actors across society in every country: governments, nongovernmental organizations, civil society, science and academia, health professionals, communities – and every individual. The health sector is challenged to learn, to understand and to promote the contributions of partner sectors to improving health and well-being. This includes understanding each partner's policy remit and existing strategic programmes, as well as its culture. As more partners emerge, smart governance must clarify the responsibilities for action in a world in which responsibility for health is universal and to which all contribute. For intersectoral collaboration to succeed, an essential ingredient is trust. Trust is built and sustained by sharing information and knowledge and by demonstrating competence, good intentions and follow-through. It can quickly be lost through opportunistic behaviour on the part of any partner(s).

A strong role for WHO

Member States and WHO working closely together and reaching out to engage other partners will be key to the success of Health 2020. Health 2020 will become the overarching regional framework for health development and an umbrella under which other regional policies, strategies and actions will be framed and nested. All existing commitments by the WHO European Region and its Member States also need to be seen in this light. A recent review of these commitments *(302)* indicates that Health 2020 may be seen as a reframing of many such commitments within a coherent and visionary approach, overcoming fragmentation and facilitating implementation. However, some issues need more attention now, such as the health of older people, the management of some noncommunicable diseases and the economic implications of health and disease. In addition, the study suggests that the mechanisms and principles underlying the implementation of complex strategies should be better defined and developed. Finally, the study proposes that new Regional Committee resolutions include a brief overview of the progress made on implementing previous commitments.

The Regional Office will continue to fulfil its constitutional role of acting as the directing and coordinating authority on international health work in the European Region. It will establish and maintain effective collaboration with many partners and provide technical assistance to countries. This means engaging broadly, increasing policy coherence by working on shared policy platforms, sharing health data sets, joining forces for surveillance, and supporting the development of new types of network and web-based cooperation. It will act as the European Region's repository of what works and will work with countries, through new types of country cooperation strategies. It will continue its work where it has a direct mandate in setting standards, such as in biological and pharmaceutical products. Close cooperation between the

WHO Regional Office for Europe, WHO headquarters and other regions will be vital.

Europe is a source of expertise and experience, particularly in the fields of health care and development, and is therefore a resource for other parts of the world. Many European countries have bilateral agencies providing technical expertise and development support. Countries across the Region contribute to, yet also benefit from, cooperation with international organizations. This resource is critical in supporting the aims of Health 2020. The role of WHO and its interrelationship with these organizations will rest not only on its pursuit of technical excellence, evidence-informed practice and results-based management but also on its commitment to work with others in helping Member States fully to realize their full health potential.

While helping to bring about this desired world, WHO is in the process of reform, designed to improve health outcomes, ensure greater coherence in global health, and create itself as an organization that pursues excellence, effectiveness, efficiency, responsiveness, transparency and accountability. Overall, the aim is to move from an organization that delivers separate outputs through a series of technical programmes to one that achieves impact, working with national authorities, through the combined and coordinated efforts of country offices, regional offices, headquarters and its outposts, all operating as part of an interdependent network.

Looking forward

In an interdependent world, the need for countries to act together becomes ever more important. Today, a complex array of global and regional forces challenges people's health and its determinants. Although more people than ever before now have the chance to attain better health, no country can harness the potential of innovation and change or resolve the challenges to health and well-being in isolation. The future prosperity of the European Region depends on its willingness and ability to seize new opportunities for the health and well-being of present and future generations.

WHO has a special role to play in pursuing the objective defined in its Constitution *(1)*: "the attainment by all peoples of the highest possible level of health". The world envisaged by WHO is one in which gaps in health outcomes are narrowed; universal access to health care is achieved; countries have resilient health systems, based on primary health care, that can meet the expectations and needs of their peoples; internationally agreed health goals are reached; noncommunicable diseases are controlled; and countries cope with disease outbreaks and natural disasters. Never before in history have the means to reach these goals been within our grasp; never before have we had so many tools and resources at hand to help attain them. Yet we have not hitherto harnessed these resources and the knowledge available to us sufficiently, so that all citizens may benefit from them.

We are particularly challenged to address health inequalities and the health of future generations. Unless we do so, there is a real risk that the health status of some groups may become worse than that of their forebears. Health 2020 is designed to help overcome some of the principal barriers that have held us back. It provides a vision, a strategic path, a set of priorities and a range of suggestions to show what works, based on research and experience in many countries. It states clearly that many partners need to come together to achieve better health and well-being. It does not imply that health is everything or the only aspect of life to be valued – societies and individuals have many goals that they wish to achieve. Nevertheless, Health 2020 emphasizes that health is crucial as a means to achieve other goals in life. Health is a resource that enables every person to realize his or her potential and to contribute to the overall development of society. Let us therefore work together to build and use this precious resource wisely and for the benefit of all.

References

1. Constitution of the World Health Organization. In: *Basic documents*. 45th ed. Supplement, October 2006. Geneva, World Health Organization, 2006 (http://www.who.int/governance/eb/who_constitution_en.pdf, accessed 21 June 2013).
2. *Universal Declaration of Human Rights*. Paris, United Nations, 1948 (http://www.un.org/en/documents/udhr, accessed 21 June 2013).
3. *International Covenant on Economic, Social and Cultural Rights*. New York, United Nations, 1966 (http://treaties.un.org/doc/Publication/MTDSG/Volume%20I/Chapter%20IV/IV-3.en.pdf, accessed 21 June 2013).
4. World Health Assembly resolution WHA30.43. In: *Handbook of resolutions and decisions of the World Health Assembly and the Executive Board. Volume II: 1978–1984*. Geneva, World Health Organization, 1985:1.
5. *Declaration of Alma-Ata. International Conference on Primary Health Care, Alma-Ata, USSR, 6–12 September 1978*. Geneva, World Health Organization, 1978 (http://www.who.int/publications/almaata_declaration_en.pdf, accessed 21 June 2013).
6. United Nations General Assembly. *Global Strategy for Health for All by the Year 2000*. New York, United Nations, 1981 (http://www.un-documents.net/a36r43.htm, accessed 21 June 2013).
7. World Health Assembly. *World Health Declaration*. Geneva, World Health Organization, 1998.
8. *Rio Political Declaration on Social Determinants of Health*. World Conference on Social Determinants of Health, Rio de Janeiro, Brazil, 21 October 2011. Geneva, World Health Organization, 2011 (http://www.who.int/sdhconference/declaration/en, accessed 21 June 2013).
9. United Nations General Assembly. *United Nations Millennium Declaration*. New York, United Nations, 2000 (http://www.un.org/millennium/declaration/ares552e.htm, accessed 21 June 2013).
10. Millennium Development Goals [web site]. New York, United Nations, 2013 (http://www.un.org/millenniumgoals, accessed 21 June 2013).
11. *Human development report 2010. The real wealth of nations*. New York, United Nations Development Programme, 2010 (http://hdr.undp.org/en/media/HDR_2010_EN_Complete_reprint.pdf, accessed 21 June 2013).
12. *Eurostat feasibility study for well-being indicators*. Brussels, Eurostat, 2010 (http://epp.eurostat.ec.europa.eu/portal/page/portal/gdp_and_beyond/documents/Feasibility_study_Well-Being_Indicators.pdf, accessed 21 June 2013).
13. *The right to health*. Geneva, Office of the United Nations High Commissioner for Human Rights, 2008 (http://www.ohchr.org/Documents/Publications/Factsheet31.pdf, accessed 21 June 2013).
14. *2005 World Summit Outcome. General Assembly resolution A/RES/60/1*. New York, United Nations, 2005 (http://unpan1.un.org/intradoc/groups/public/documents/un/unpan021752.pdf, accessed 21 June 2013).
15. *European Social Charter (revised)*. Strasbourg, Council of Europe, 1996 (http://conventions.coe.int/Treaty/en/Treaties/Html/163.htm, accessed 21 June 2013).

16. *Charter of Fundamental Rights of the European Union*. Brussels, Commission of the European Communities, 2010 (Official Journal of the European Communities, 2000/C 364/01A, http://www.europarl.europa.eu/charter/pdf/text_en.pdf, accessed 21 June 2013).

17. *European review of social determinants of health and the health divide*. Copenhagen, WHO Regional Office for Europe (forthcoming).

18. *Roma and Travellers glossary*. Strasbourg, Council of Europe, 2006.

19. Sadler JZ et al. Can medicalization be good? Situating medicalization within bioethics. *Theoretical Medical and Bioethics*, 2009, 30:411–425.

20. WHO Framework Convention on Tobacco Control [web site]. Geneva, World Health Organization, 2013 (http://www.who.int/fctc/en/index.html, accessed 21 June 2013).

21. United Nations General Assembly. *Resolution A/RES/64/108 on global health and foreign policy*. New York, United Nations, 2009 (http://www.un.org/en/ga/64/resolutions.shtml, accessed 21 June 2013).

22. *White paper. Together for health: a strategic approach for the EU 2008–2013*. Brussels, Commission of the European Communities, 2007 (COM(2007) 630 final; http://ec.europa.eu/health/ph_overview/Documents/strategy_wp_en.pdf, accessed 21 June 2013).

23. *The Health for All policy framework for the WHO European Region: 2005 update*. Copenhagen, WHO Regional Office for Europe, 2005 (document EUR/RC55/8, http://www.euro.who.int/__data/assets/pdf_file/0005/87881/RC55_edoc08.pdf, accessed 21 June 2013).

24. *Health Systems, Health and Wealth: WHO European Ministerial Conference on Health Systems: Tallinn, Estonia, 25–27 June 2008: report*. Copenhagen, WHO Regional Office for Europe, 2009 (http://www.euro.who.int/__data/assets/pdf_file/0006/78918/E92150.pdf, accessed 21 June 2013).

25. *The European health report 2012: charting the way to well-being*. Copenhagen, WHO Regional Office for Europe, 2013 (http://www.euro.who.int/en/what-we-do/data-and-evidence/european-health-report-2012, accessed 21 June 2013).

26. European Health for All database [online database]. Copenhagen, WHO Regional Office for Europe, 2013 (http://data.euro.who.int/hfadb, accessed 21 June 2013).

27. Commission on Social Determinants of Health. *Closing the gap in a generation: health equity through action on the social determinants of health. Final report of the Commission on Social Determinants of Health*. Geneva, World Health Organization, 2008 (http://www.who.int/social_determinants/resources/gkn_lee_al.pdf, accessed 21 June 2013).

28. *United Nations Framework Convention on Climate Change*. New York, United Nations, 1992 (http://unfccc.int/resource/docs/convkp/conveng.pdf, accessed 21 June 2013).

29. Dooris M et al. The settings-based approach to health promotion. In: Tsouros A et al., eds. *Health-promoting universities: concept, experience and framework for action*. Copenhagen, WHO Regional Office for Europe, 1998.

30. *Ottawa Charter for Health Promotion*. Copenhagen, WHO Regional Office for Europe, 1986 (http://www.euro.who.int/en/who-we-are/policy-documents/ottawa-charter-for-health-promotion,-1986, accessed 21 June 2013).

31. *Interim first report on social determinants of health and the health divide in the WHO European Region – executive summary*. Copenhagen, WHO Regional Office for Europe, 2010 (http://www.euro.who.int/__data/assets/pdf_file/0003/124464/E94370.pdf, accessed 21 June 2013).

32. Adler NE et al. Socioeconomic status and health: the challenge of the gradient. *American Psychologist*, 1994,49:15–24.
33. *Genome-based research and population health. Report of an expert workshop held at the Rockefeller Foundation Study and Conference Centre, Bellagio, Italy, 14–20 April 2005*. Cambridge, PHG Foundation, 2005.
34. Wertz D, Fletcher JC, Berg K *Review of ethical issues in medical genetics. Report of consultants to WHO*. Geneva, World Health Organization, 2003.
35. Kirschner MW. The meaning of systems biology. *Cell*, 2005, 121:503–504.
36. McDaid D, Sassi F, Merkur S, eds. *Promoting health, preventing disease: the economic case*. Maidenhead, Open University Press (forthcoming).
37. Stuckler D, Basu S, McKee M. Budget crises, health, and social welfare programs. *British Medical Journal*, 2010, 340:c3311.
38. Rittel H, Webber M. Dilemmas in a general theory of planning. *Policy Sciences*, 1973, 4:155–169.
39. *Tackling wicked problems: a public policy perspective*. Canberra, Australian Public Service Commission, 2007.
40. Dahlgren G, Whitehead M. *Tackling inequalities in health: what can we learn from what has been tried?* London, King's Fund, 1993.
41. *Interim second report on social determinants of health and the health divide in the WHO European Region*. Copenhagen, WHO Regional Office for Europe, 2011 (http://www.euro.who.int/__data/assets/pdf_file/0010/148375/id5E_2ndRepSocialDet-jh.pdf, accessed 21 June 2013).
42. *Reducing health inequalities in the EU. European Parliament Resolution, 9 March 2011*. Brussels, European Parliament, 2011 (http://www.europarl.europa.eu/sides/getDoc.do?type=REPORT&reference=A7-2011-0032&language=EN, accessed 21 June 2013).
43. *The Banja Luka Pledge. Health in all policies in south-eastern Europe: a shared goal and responsibility. Third Health Ministers' Forum, Banja Luka, Bosnia and Herzegovina, 13–14 October 2011*. Copenhagen, WHO Regional Office for Europe, 2011 (http://www.euro.who.int/__data/assets/pdf_file/0020/152471/e95832.pdf, accessed 21 June 2013).
44. Wilkinson R, Pickett K. *The spirit level: why more equal societies almost always do better*. London, Allen Lane, 2009.
45. Popay J et al. *Understanding and tackling social exclusion. Final report to the WHO Commission on Social Determinants of Health, from the Social Exclusion Knowledge Network*. Lancaster, WHO Social Exclusion Knowledge Network, 2008 (http://www.who.int/social_determinants/knowledge_networks/final_reports/sekn_final%20report_042008.pdf, accessed 21 June 2013).
46. The Marmot Review. *Fair society, healthy lives: strategic review of health inequalities in England 2010. London, Marmot Review, 2010* (http://www.ucl.ac.uk/marmotreview, accessed 21 June 2013).
47. *World Health Assembly resolution WHA62.14 on reducing health inequities through action on the social determinants of health*. Geneva, World Health Organization, 2009.
48. *Interim report on implementation of the Tallinn Charter*. Copenhagen, WHO Regional Office for Europe, 2010 (http://www.euro.who.int/__data/assets/pdf_file/0019/134470/08E_InterimTallinn_110515-V2.pdf, accessed 21 June 2013).

49. *Governance and delivery for social determinants. Task group report, European review on social determinants of health*. Copenhagen, WHO Regional Office for Europe (in press).

50. Marmot M et al. Building of the global movement for health equity: from Santiago to Rio and beyond. *Lancet*, 2011, 379:181–188.

51. Kickbusch I, Gleicher D. *Governance for health in the 21st century*. Copenhagen, WHO Regional Office for Europe, 2012 (http://www.euro.who.int/__data/assets/pdf_file/0019/171334/RC62BD01-Governance-for-Health-Web.pdf, accessed 21 June 2013).

52. Worldwide Governance Indicators Project [web site]. Washington, DC, World Bank, 2013 (http://info.worldbank.org/governance/wgi/resources.htm, accessed 21 June 2013).

53. Marteau TM et al. Judging nudging: can nudging improve population health? *British Medical Journal*, 2011, 342:d228.

54. Nanda G et al. *Accelerating progress towards achieving the MDG to improve maternal health: a collection of promising approaches*. Washington, DC, World Bank, 2005.

55. *Unsafe abortion: global and regional estimates of the incidence of unsafe abortion and associated mortality in 2008*. 6th ed. Geneva, World Health Organization, 2011 (http://www.who.int/reproductivehealth/publications/unsafe_abortion/9789241501118/en, accessed 21 June 2013).

56. Sedgh G et al. Induced abortion: rates and trends worldwide. *Lancet*, 2007, 370:1338–1345.

57. Oliveira da Silva M et al. The reproductive health report. The state of sexual and reproductive health within the European Union. *European Journal of Contraception and Reproductive Health Care,* 2011, 16(Suppl. 1).

58. Currie C et al. *Inequalities in young people's health. Health behaviour in school-aged children. International report from the 2005/2006 survey*. Copenhagen, WHO Regional Office for Europe, 2008 (http://www.euro.who.int/__data/assets/pdf_file/0005/53852/E91416.pdf, accessed 21 June 2013).

59. Malarcher S. *Social determinants of sexual and reproductive health. Informing future research and programme implementation*. Geneva, World Health Organization, 2010 (http://www.who.int/reproductivehealth/publications/social_science/9789241599528/en/index.html, accessed 21 June 2013).

60. *Children: reducing mortality*. Geneva, World Health Organization, 2012 (Fact sheet No. 178; http://www.who.int/mediacentre/factsheets/fs178/en/index.html, accessed 21 June 2013).

61. *Newborns: reducing mortality*. Geneva, World Health Organization, 2012 (Fact sheet No. 333; http://www.who.int/mediacentre/factsheets/fs333/en/index.html, accessed 21 June 2013).

62. Beck S et al. The worldwide incidence of preterm birth: a systematic review of maternal mortality and morbidity. *Bulletin of the World Health Organization*, 2010, 88:31–38.

63. Effective perinatal care training package (EPC) [web site]. Copenhagen, WHO Regional Office for Europe, 2013 (http://www.euro.who.int/en/what-we-do/health-topics/Life-stages/maternal-and-newborn-health/policy-and-tools/effective-perinatal-care-training-package-epc, accessed 21 June 2013).

64. WHO, UNICEF, UNFPA and World Bank. *Trends in maternal mortality: 1990 to 2008. Estimates developed by WHO, UNICEF, UNFPA and the World Bank*. Geneva, World Health Organization, 2010 (http://www.who.int/reproductivehealth/publications/monitoring/9789241500265/en/index.html, accessed 21 June 2013).

65. Statistics and stories: improving the quality of maternal and neonatal health in Europe. *Entre Nous: the European Magazine for Sexual and Reproductive Health*, 2010, 70 (http://www.euro.who.int/__data/assets/pdf_file/0013/123016/en70.pdf, accessed 21 June 2013).

66. Are we on track? Progress towards MDG3, 4 and 5 in Europe. *Entre Nous: the European Magazine for Sexual and Reproductive Health*, 2011, 71 (http://www.euro.who.int/__data/assets/pdf_file/0016/132208/en71.pdf, accessed 21 June 2013).

67. *European strategic approach for making pregnancy safer: improving maternal and perinatal health*. Copenhagen, WHO Regional Office for Europe, 2009 (http://www.euro.who.int/__data/assets/pdf_file/0012/98796/E90771.pdf, accessed 21 June 2013).

68. *How health systems can accelerate progress towards Millennium Development Goals 4 and 5 on child and maternal health by promoting gender equity*. Copenhagen, WHO Regional Office for Europe, 2010 (http://www.euro.who.int/__data/assets/pdf_file/0006/127527/e94498.pdf, accessed 21 June 2013).

69. *Millennium Development Goals in the WHO European Region: a situational analysis at the eve of the five-year countdown*. Copenhagen, WHO Regional Office for Europe, 2010 (http://www.euro.who.int/__data/assets/pdf_file/0003/87438/E93723.pdf, accessed 21 June 2013).

70. *The European health report 2009 – Health and health systems*. Copenhagen, WHO Regional Office for Europe, 2009 (http://www.euro.who.int/document/e93103.pdf, accessed 21 June 2013).

71. *A review of progress in maternal health in eastern Europe and central Asia*. Istanbul, UNFPA Regional Office for Eastern Europe and Central Asia, 2009.

72. *Achieving Millennium Development Goal 5: target 5A and 5B on reducing maternal mortality and achieving universal access to reproductive health. Briefing note*. Geneva, World Health Organization, 2009 (http://www.who.int/reproductivehealth/publications/monitoring/rhr_09_06/en/index.html, accessed 21 June 2013).

73. World Health Organization, United Nations Population Fund, UNICEF and World Bank. *Accelerated implementation of maternal and newborn continuum of care as part of improving reproductive health: mapping of in-country activities. Joint country support*. Geneva, World Health Organization, 2009 (http://www.who.int/reproductivehealth/publications/monitoring/9789241599733/en, accessed 21 June 2013).

74. *Reproductive health strategy to accelerate progress towards the attainment of international development goals and targets*. Geneva, World Health Organization, 2004 (http://www.who.int/reproductivehealth/publications/general/RHR_04_8/en, accessed 21 June 2013).

75. *WHO regional strategy on sexual and reproductive health*. Copenhagen, WHO Regional Office for Europe, 2001 (http://www.euro.who.int/__data/assets/pdf_file/0004/69529/e74558.pdf, accessed 21 June 2013).

76. *Global strategy for the prevention and control of sexually transmitted infections: 2006–2015. Breaking the chain of transmission*. Geneva, World Health Organization, 2007 (http://www.who.int/reproductivehealth/publications/rtis/9789241563475/en/index.html, accessed 21 June 2013).

77. WHO and UNICEF. *Global strategy for infant and young child feeding*. Geneva, World Health Organization, 2003 (http://www.who.int/child_adolescent_health/documents/9241562218/en/index.html, accessed 21 June 2013).

78. *The MDGs in Europe and central Asia: achievements, challenges and the way forward.* Geneva, United Nations Economic Commission for Europe, 2010 (http://www.unece.org/commission/MDGs/2010_MDG.pdf, accessed 21 June 2013).

79. United Nations Secretary-General. *Global Strategy for Women's and Children's Health.* Geneva, Partnership for Maternal, Newborn and Child Health, 2010 (http://www.who.int/pmnch/activities/jointactionplan/en/index.html, accessed 21 June 2013).

80. Commission on Information and Accountability for Women's and Children's Health. *Keeping promises, measuring results.* Geneva, World Health Organization, 2011 (http://www.who.int/topics/millennium_development_goals/accountability_commission/en, accessed 21 June 2013).

81. *WHO's role in the follow-up to the United Nations High-level Plenary Meeting of the General Assembly on the Millennium Development Goals.* Geneva, World Health Organization, 2011 (resolution WHA64.12; http://apps.who.int/gb/or/e/e_wha64r1.html, accessed 21 June 2013).

82. *World health statistics 2011.* Geneva, World Health Organization, 2011 (http://www.who.int/whosis/whostat/EN_WHS2011_Full.pdf, accessed 21 June 2013).

83. *Children's Environment and Health Action Plan for Europe. Fourth Ministerial Conference on Environment and Health, Budapest, Hungary, 23–25 June 2004.* Copenhagen, WHO Regional Office for Europe, 2004 (http://www.euro.who.int/document/e83338.pdf, accessed 21 June 2013).

84. *Countdown to 2015: tracking progress in maternal, newborn & child survival. The 2008 report.* Geneva, World Health Organization, 2008 (http://www.who.int/child_adolescent_health/documents/9789280642841/en/index.html, accessed 21 June 2013).

85. *European Charter on Counteracting Obesity.* Copenhagen, WHO Regional Office for Europe, 2006 (http://www.euro.who.int/__data/assets/pdf_file/0009/87462/E89567.pdf, accessed 21 June 2013).

86. Patton GC et al. Global patterns of mortality in young people: a systematic analysis of population health data. *Lancet*, 2009, 374:881–892.

87. *Youth-friendly health policies and services in the European Region.* Copenhagen, WHO Regional Office for Europe, 2010 (http://www.euro.who.int/__data/assets/pdf_file/0017/123128/E94322.pdf, accessed 21 June 2013).

88. *Mental health: facing the challenges, building solutions. Report from the WHO European Ministerial Conference.* Copenhagen, WHO Regional Office for Europe, 2005 (http://www.euro.who.int/document/E87301.pdf, accessed 21 June 2013).

89. Sethi D, Racioppi F, Mitis F. *Youth and road safety in Europe: policy briefing.* Copenhagen, WHO Regional Office for Europe, 2007 (http://www.euro.who.int/__data/assets/pdf_file/0003/98454/E90142.pdf, accessed 21 June 2013).

90. *European report on child injury prevention.* Copenhagen, WHO Regional Office for Europe, 2008 (http://www.euro.who.int/__data/assets/pdf_file/0003/83757/E92049.pdf, accessed 21 June 2013).

91. "Young people's health as a whole-of-society response" series [web site]. Copenhagen, WHO Regional Office for Europe, 2009 (http://www.euro.who.int/en/what-we-do/health-topics/Life-stages/child-and-adolescent-health/publications/2013/young-peoples-health-as-a-whole-of-society-response-series, accessed 21 June 2013).

92. *European strategy for child and adolescent health and development*. Copenhagen, WHO Regional Office for Europe, 2005 (http://www.euro.who.int/__data/assets/pdf_file/0020/79400/E87710.pdf, accessed 21 June 2013).

93. *Adolescent-friendly health services – an agenda for change*. Geneva, World Health Organization, 2002 (http://www.who.int/maternal_child_adolescent/documents/fch_cah_02_14/en/index.html, accessed 21 June 2013).

94. *Youth and health risks. Report by the Secretariat*. Geneva, World Health Organization, 2011 (document A64/25; http://apps.who.int/gb/ebwha/pdf_files/WHA64/A64_R28-en.pdf, accessed 21 June 2013).

95. *Helping parents in developing countries improve adolescents' health*. Geneva, World Health Organization, 2007 (http://www.who.int/maternal_child_adolescent/documents/9789241595841/en/index.html, accessed 21 June 2013).

96. *The European health report 2005 – Public health action for healthier children and populations*. Copenhagen, WHO Regional Office for Europe, 2005 (http://www.euro.who.int/document/e87325.pdf, accessed 21 June 2013).

97. *A critical link: interventions for physical growth and psychological development*. Geneva, World Health Organization, 1999 (http://www.who.int/child_adolescent_health/documents/chs_cah_99_3/en/index.html, accessed 21 June 2013).

98. *Early child development: a powerful equalizer. Final report to WHO Commission on Social Determinants of Health*. Geneva, World Health Organization, 2007 (http://www.who.int/child_adolescent_health/documents/ecd_final_m30/en/index.html, accessed 21 June 2013).

99. The *Lancet* child development in developing countries series [web site]. Geneva, World Health Organization, 2007 (http://www.who.int/child_adolescent_health/documents/lancet_child_development/en/index.html, accessed 21 June 2013).

100. *IMCI care for development: for the healthy growth and development of children*. Geneva, World Health Organization, 2001 (http://www.who.int/maternal_child_adolescent/documents/imci_care_for_development/en/index.html, accessed 21 June 2013).

101. *The European report on tobacco control policy*. Copenhagen, WHO Regional Office for Europe, 2002 (http://www.euro.who.int/__data/assets/pdf_file/0007/68065/E74573.pdf, accessed 21 June 2013).

102. *The challenge of obesity in the WHO European Region and the strategies for response*. Copenhagen, WHO Regional Office for Europe, 2007 (http://www.euro.who.int/__data/assets/pdf_file/0010/74746/E90711.pdf, accessed 21 June 2013).

103. *Childhood obesity surveillance in the European Region*. Copenhagen, WHO Regional Office for Europe, 2009 (Fact sheet 5; http://www.euro.who.int/__data/assets/pdf_file/0020/123176/FactSheet_5.pdf, accessed 21 June 2013).

104. *Integrated Management of Childhood Illness computerized training tool*. Geneva, World Health Organization, 2012 (http://www.icatt-training.org, accessed 21 June 2013).

105. *IMCI chart booklet – standard*. Geneva, World Health Organization, 2008 (http://www.who.int/child_adolescent_health/documents/IMCI_chartbooklet/en/index.html, accessed 21 June 2013).

106. *Joint statement by heads of United Nations entities for the launch of the International Year of Youth*. New York, United Nations, 2011 (http://social.un.org/youthyear/docs/iyyjointstatement.pdf, accessed 21 June 2013).

107. *Broadening the horizon: balancing protection and risk for adolescents*. Geneva, World Health Organization, 2001 (http://www.who.int/child_adolescent_health/documents/fch_cah_01_20/en/index.html, accessed 21 June 2013).

108. *A guide for population-based approaches to increasing levels of physical activity: implementation of the WHO global strategy on diet, physical activity and health*. Geneva, World Health Organization, 2007 (http://www.who.int/dietphysicalactivity, accessed 21 June 2013).

109. WHO and UNICEF. *Child and adolescent injury prevention: a global call to action*. Geneva, World Health Organization, 2005 (http://whqlibdoc.who.int/publications/2005/9241593415_eng.pdf, accessed 21 June 2013).

110. *WHO European strategy for child and adolescent health and development: from resolution to action 2005–2008*. Copenhagen, WHO Regional Office for Europe, 2008 (http://www.euro.who.int/__data/assets/pdf_file/0003/81831/E91655.pdf, accessed 21 June 2013).

111. Stuckler D et al. The public health effect of economic crises and alternative policy responses in Europe: an empirical analysis. *Lancet*, 2009, 374:315–323.

112. Consolidated version of the Treaty on the Functioning of the European Union. *Official Journal of the European Union*, 2008, C 115/47(9 May) (http://eur-lex.europa.eu/LexUriServ/LexUriServ.do?uri=OJ:C:2008:115:0047:0199:en:PDF, accessed 21 June 2013).

113. World Health Assembly resolution 60.25. *Strategy for integrating gender analysis and actions in the work of WHO*. Geneva, World Health Organization, 2007, (http://www.who.int/gender/documents/gender/who_fch_gwh_08_1/en, accessed 21 June 2013).

114. Huber M et al. *Facts and figures on long-term care – Europe and North America*. Vienna, European Centre for Social Welfare Policy and Research, 2009.

115. Przywar B. *Projecting future health care expenditure at European level: drivers, methodology and main results*. Brussels, European Commission, 2010 (European Economic Papers No. 417).

116. Huber M et al. *Quality in and equality of access to healthcare services*. Brussels, European Commission, 2008.

117. *Strategy and action plan for healthy ageing in Europe, 2012–2020*. Copenhagen, WHO Regional Office for Europe, 2012 (http://www.euro.who.int/__data/assets/pdf_file/0008/175544/RC62wd10Rev1-Eng.pdf, accessed 21 June 2013).

118. *How can health systems respond to population ageing?* Copenhagen, WHO Regional Office for Europe, 2009 (http://www.euro.who.int/__data/assets/pdf_file/0004/64966/E92560.pdf, accessed 21 June 2013).

119. *Palliative care: the solid facts*. Copenhagen, WHO Regional Office for Europe, 2004 (http://www.euro.who.int/__data/assets/pdf_file/0003/98418/E82931.pdf, accessed 21 June 2013).

120. Hall S et al. *Palliative care for older people: better practices*. Copenhagen, WHO Regional Office for Europe, 2011 (http://www.euro.who.int/en/what-we-publish/abstracts/palliative-care-for-older-people-better-practices, accessed 21 June 2013).

121. World Health Assembly resolution WHA52.7 on active ageing. In: *Fifty-second World Health Assembly, Geneva, 17–25 May 1999. Volume 1*. Resolutions and decisions, annexes. Geneva, World Health Organization, 1999:8–9.

122. *WHO Executive Board resolution EB130.R6 on strengthening noncommunicable disease policies to promote active ageing*. Geneva, World Health Organization, 2012 (http://apps.who.int/gb/ebwha/pdf_files/EB130/B130_R6-en.pdf, accessed 21 June 2013).

123. United Nations/DESA. *The Madrid International Plan of Action on Ageing*. New York, United Nations, 2002.

124. *Active ageing: a policy framework*. Geneva, World Health Organization, 2002 (http://www.who.int/ageing/publications/active/en, accessed 21 June 2013).

125. Van Liemt G. *Human trafficking in Europe: an economic perspective*. Declaration/WP/31/2004. Geneva, International Labour Organization, 2004.

126. *How health systems can address health inequalities linked to migration and ethnicity*. Copenhagen, WHO Regional Office for Europe, 2010 (http://www.euro.who.int/__data/assets/pdf_file/0005/127526/e94497.pdf, accessed 21 June 2013).

127. Carballo M. Non-communicable diseases. In: Fernandes A, Pereira Miguel J, eds. *Health and migration in the European Union: better health for all in an inclusive society*. Lisbon, Instituto Nacional de Saúde Doutor Ricardo Jorge, 2009:71–78 (http://www.insa.pt/sites/INSA/Portugues/Publicacoes/Outros/Paginas/HealthMigrationEU2.aspx, accessed 21 June 2013).

128. Carballo M. Communicable diseases. In: Fernandes A, Pereira Miguel J, eds. *Health and migration in the European Union: better health for all in an inclusive society*. Lisbon, Instituto Nacional de Saúde Doutor Ricardo Jorge, 2009:53–69 (http://www.insa.pt/sites/INSA/Portugues/Publicacoes/Outros/Paginas/HealthMigrationEU2.aspx, accessed 21 June 2013).

129. Carta MG et al. Migration and mental health in Europe (the State of the Mental Health in Europe Working Group: Appendix 1). *Clinical Practice and Epidemiology in Mental Health*, 2005, 1:13.

130. *Migrant health: background note to the ECDC report on migration and infectious diseases in the EU*. Stockholm, European Centre for Disease Prevention and Control, 2009 (http://www.ecdc.europa.eu/en/publications/Publications/0907_TER_Migrant_health_Background_note.pdf, accessed 21 June 2013).

131. *An EU framework for national Roma integration strategies up to 2020*. Brussels, European Commission, 2011 (http://ec.europa.eu/justice/policies/discrimination/docs/com_2011_173_en.pdf, accessed 21 June 2013).

132. *The Roma in central and eastern Europe: avoiding the dependency trap*. Bratislava, United Nations Development Programme, 2003 (http://www.arab-hdr.org/publications/other/undp/hdr/regional/avoiding-dep-trap-03e.pdf, accessed 21 June 2013).

133. *Health and the Roma community, analysis of the situation in Europe*. Madrid, Fundación Secretariado Gitano, 2009 (http://ec.europa.eu/social/BlobServlet?docId=4309&langId=en, accessed 21 June 2013).

134. Schaaf M. *Confronting a hidden disease: TB in Roma communities*. New York, Open Society Institute, 2007 (http://www.soros.org/initiatives/health/focus/roma/articles_publications/publications/confronting_20070206/confronting_20070122.pdf, accessed 21 June 2013).

135. *Left out: Roma and access to health care in eastern and south-eastern Europe*. New York, Open Society Institute, 2007 (http://www.romadecade.org/files/downloads/Health%20Resources/leftout_20070423.pdf, accessed 21 June 2013).

136. *At risk: Roma and the displaced in southeast Europe*. Bratislava, United Nations Development Programme, 2006 (http://europeandcis.undp.org/home/show/A3C29ADB-F203-1EE9-BB0A277C80C5F9F2, accessed 21 June 2013).

137. Milcher S. Poverty and the determinants of welfare for Roma and other vulnerable groups in southeastern Europe. *Comparative Economic Studies*, 2006, 48:20–35 (http://europeandcis.undp.org/files/uploads/_rbec%20web/roma%20portal/susanne.pdf, accessed 21 June 2013).

138. *Republic of Macedonia, Multiple Indicator Cluster Survey 2005–2006*. Skopje, State Statistical Office, the former Yugoslav Republic of Macedonia, 2007 (http://www.unicef.org/tfyrmacedonia/MICS-ENG-1(1).pdf, accessed 21 June 2013).

139. *The state of children in Serbia in 2006*. Belgrade, UNICEF, 2007 (http://www.unicef.org/serbia/State_of_Children_in_Serbia_2006_1-56.pdf, accessed 21 June 2013).

140. *First findings of Roma Task Force and report on social inclusion*. Brussels, European Commission, 2010 (http://europa.eu/rapid/pressReleasesAction.do?reference=MEMO/10/701&type=HTML, accessed 21 June 2013).

141. *WHO Regional Committee for Europe resolution EUR/RC52/R7 on poverty and health – evidence and action in WHO's European Region*. Copenhagen, WHO Regional Office for Europe, 2002 (http://www.euro.who.int/__data/assets/pdf_file/0012/117111/R07.23598ema.pdf, accessed 21 June 2013).

142. *World Health Assembly resolution WHA61.17 on health of migrants*. Geneva, World Health Organization, 2008 (http://apps.who.int/gb/ebwha/pdf_files/WHA61-REC1/A61_REC1-en.pdf, accessed 21 June 2013).

143. *Health of migrants – the way forward. Report of a global consultation*. Madrid, Spain, 3–5 March 2010. Geneva, World Health Organization, 2010 (http://www.who.int/hac/events/consultation_report_health_migrants_colour_web.pdf, accessed 21 June 2013).

144. *Bratislava Declaration on Health, Human Rights and Migration*. Strasbourg, Council of Europe, 2007 (http://www.coe.int/t/dg3/health%5CSource%5Cdeclaration_en.pdf, accessed 21 June 2013).

145. *Recommendation CM/REC(2011)13 of the Committee of Ministers to Member States on mobility, migration and access to health care*. Strasbourg, Council of Europe, 2011 (http://bit.ly/rKs2YD, accessed 21 June 2013).

146. *International Convention on the Protection of the Rights of All Migrant Workers and Members of Their Families*. Geneva, Office of the United Nations High Commissioner for Human Rights, 1990 (http://www2.ohchr.org/english/law/cmw.htm, accessed 21 June 2013).

147. *Council conclusions on an EU Framework for National Roma Integration Strategies up to 2020*. Brussels, Council of the European Union, 2011 (http://www.consilium.europa.eu/uedocs/cms_data/docs/pressdata/en/lsa/122100.pdf, accessed 21 June 2013).

148. Payne S. *How can gender equity be addressed through health systems?* Copenhagen, WHO Regional Office for Europe, 2009 (http://www.euro.who.int/__data/assets/pdf_file/0006/64941/E92846.pdf, accessed 21 June 2013).

149. *Youth and health risks. Resolution WHA64.28*, 24 May 2011. Geneva, World Health Organization, 2011.

150. Green G, Tsouros A, eds. *City leadership for health. Summary evaluation of Phase IV of the WHO European Healthy Cities Network*. Copenhagen, WHO Regional Office for Europe, 2008 (http://www.euro.who.int/__data/assets/pdf_file/0004/98257/E91886.pdf, accessed 21 June 2013).

151. *Help wanted? Providing and paying for long-term care*. Paris, Organisation for Economic Co-operation and Development, 2011.

152. Defining civil society [web site]. Washington, DC, World Bank, 2010 (http://web.worldbank.org/WBSITE/EXTERNAL/TOPICS/CSO/0,,contentMDK:20101499~menuPK:244752~-pagePK:220503~piPK:220476~theSitePK:228717,00.html, accessed 21 June 2013).

153. *Progress made in the implementation of the Declaration of Commitment on HIV/AIDS and the Political Declaration on HIV/AIDS. Report by the Secretary-General.* New York, United Nations, 2009 (http://data.unaids.org/pub/Report/2009/20090616_sg_report_ga_progress_en.pdf, accessed 21 June 2013).

154. Chapman DP, Perry GS, Strine TW. The vital link between chronic disease and depressive disorders. *Prevention of Chronic Diseases*, 2005, 2 (http://www.cdc.gov/pcd/issues/2005/jan/04_0066.htm, accessed 21 June 2013).

155. *European cardiovascular disease statistics 2008*. Brussels, European Heart Network, 2008 (http://www.ehnheart.org/cvd-statistics.html, accessed 21 June 2013).

156. Suhrcke M et al. *Chronic disease: an economic perspective*. London, Oxford Health Alliance, 2006.

157. Bloom DE et al. *The global economic burden of noncommunicable diseases.* Geneva, World Economic Forum, 2011 (http://www3.weforum.org/docs/WEF_Harvard_HE_GlobalEconomicBurdenNonCommunicableDiseases_2011.pdf, accessed 21 June 2013).

158. *European Strategy for Tobacco Control*. Copenhagen, WHO Regional Office for Europe, 2002 (http://www.euro.who.int/__data/assets/pdf_file/0016/68101/E77976.pdf, accessed 21 June 2013).

159. *European Action Plan for Food and Nutrition Policy 2007–2012*. Copenhagen, WHO Regional Office for Europe, 2008 (http://www.euro.who.int/__data/assets/pdf_file/0017/74402/E91153.pdf, accessed 21 June 2013).

160. *Framework for alcohol policy in the WHO European Region*. Copenhagen, WHO Regional Office for Europe, 2005 (http://www.euro.who.int/__data/assets/pdf_file/0007/79396/E88335.pdf, accessed 21 June 2013).

161. *Steps to health. A European framework to promote physical activity for health*. Copenhagen, WHO Regional Office for Europe, 2007 (http://www.euro.who.int/__data/assets/pdf_file/0020/101684/E90191.pdf, accessed 21 June 2013).

162. MPOWER [web site]. Geneva, World Health Organization, 2013 (http://www.who.int/tobacco/mpower/en, accessed 21 June 2013).

163. Raise taxes on tobacco [web site]. Geneva, World Health Organization, 2013 (http://www.who.int/tobacco/mpower/raise_taxes/en/index.html, accessed 21 June 2013).

164. *Global strategy to reduce the harmful use of alcohol*. Geneva, World Health Organization, 2010 (http://www.who.int/substance_abuse/activities/gsrhua/en/index.html, accessed 21 June 2013).

165. Cavill N, Kahlmeier S, Racioppi F, eds. *Physical activity and health in Europe*. Copenhagen, WHO Regional Office for Europe, 2006 (http://www.euro.who.int/__data/assets/pdf_file/0011/87545/E89490.pdf, accessed 21 June 2013).

166. *Promoting sport and enhancing health in European Union countries: a policy content analysis to support action*. Copenhagen, WHO Regional Office for Europe, 2011 (http://www.euro.who.int/__data/assets/pdf_file/0006/147237/e95168.pdf, accessed 21 June 2013).

167. *Global recommendations on physical activity and health*. Geneva, World Health Organization, 2010 (http://whqlibdoc.who.int/publications/2010/9789241599979_eng.pdf, accessed 21 June 2013).

168. Edwards P, Tsouros AD. *Promoting physical activity and active living in urban environments: the role of local governments. The solid facts*. Copenhagen, WHO Regional Office for Europe, 2006 (http://www.euro.who.int/__data/assets/pdf_file/0009/98424/E89498.pdf, accessed 21 June 2013).

169. *Global Strategy on Diet, Physical Activity and Health*. Geneva, World Health Organization, 2004 (http://www.who.int/dietphysicalactivity/strategy/eb11344/strategy_english_web.pdf, accessed 21 June 2013).

170. Davey Smith G et al. Genetic epidemiology and public health: hope, hype and future prospects. *Lancet*, 2005, 366:1484–1498.

171. Hall WD, Mathews R, Morley KI. Being more realistic about the public health impact of genomic medicine. *PLoS Medicine*, 2010, 7:e1000347.

172. Braubach M, Jacobs DE, Ormandy D. *Environmental burden of disease associated with inadequate housing. Methods for quantifying health impacts of selected housing risks in the WHO European Region. Summary report*. Copenhagen, WHO Regional Office for Europe, 2011 (http://www.euro.who.int/__data/assets/pdf_file/0017/145511/e95004sum.pdf, accessed 21 June 2013).

173. *WHO guidelines for indoor air quality: selected pollutants*. Copenhagen, WHO Regional Office for Europe, 2010 (http://www.euro.who.int/__data/assets/pdf_file/0009/128169/e94535.pdf, accessed 21 June 2013).

174. *Early detection. Cancer control: knowledge into action. WHO guide for effective programmes, module 3*. Geneva, World Health Organization, 2007 (http://www.who.int/cancer/modules/Early%20Detection%20Module%203.pdf, accessed 21 June 2013).

175. *Prevention of cardiovascular disease: guidelines for assessment and management of total cardiovascular risk*. Geneva, World Health Organization, 2007 (http://www.who.int/cardiovascular_diseases/guidelines/Full%20text.pdf, accessed 21 June 2013).

176. *Moscow Declaration on Healthy Lifestyles and Noncommunicable Disease Control*. Geneva, World Health Organization, 2011 (http://www.un.org/en/ga/president/65/issues/moscow_declaration_en.pdf, accessed 21 June 2013).

177. *World Health Assembly resolution WHA64.11: Preparations for the High-level Meeting of the United Nations General Assembly on the Prevention and Control of Non-communicable Diseases, following on the Moscow Conference*. Geneva, World Health Organization, 2011 (http://apps.who.int/gb/ebwha/pdf_files/WHA64-REC1/A64_REC1-en.pdf#page=21, accessed 21 June 2013).

178. *Action plan for implementation of the European Strategy for the Prevention and Control of Noncommunicable Diseases 2012–2016*. Copenhagen, WHO Regional Office for Europe, 2011 (http://www.euro.who.int/__data/assets/pdf_file/0003/147729/wd12E_NCDs_111360_revision.pdf, accessed 21 June 2013).

179. *European action plan to reduce the harmful use of alcohol 2012–2020*. Copenhagen, WHO Regional Office for Europe, 2011 (http://www.euro.who.int/__data/assets/pdf_file/0006/147732/RC61_wd13E_Alcohol_111372_ver2012.pdf, accessed 21 June 2013).

180. United Nations General Assembly. *Political Declaration of the High-level Meeting of the General Assembly on the Prevention and Control of Non-communicable Diseases*. New York, United Nations, 2011 (http://www.un.org/ga/search/view_doc.asp?symbol=A/66/L.1, accessed 21 June 2013).

181. *Preventing chronic diseases: a vital investment*. Geneva, World Health Organization, 2005 (http://www.who.int/chp/chronic_disease_report/contents/foreword.pdf, accessed 21 June 2013).

182. *The world health report 2002 – Reducing risks, promoting healthy life*. Geneva, World Health Organization, 2002 (http://www.who.int/whr/2002/en/whr02_en.pdf, accessed 21 June 2013).

183. *Gaining health. The European Strategy for the Prevention and Control of Noncommunicable Diseases*. Copenhagen, WHO Regional Office for Europe, 2006 (http://www.euro.who.int/__data/assets/pdf_file/0008/76526/E89306.pdf, accessed 21 June 2013).

184. Beaglehole R et al. Priority actions for the non-communicable disease crisis. *Lancet*, 2011, 377:1438–1447.

185. World Economic Forum and WHO. *From burden to "best buys": reducing the economic impact of non-communicable diseases in low- and middle-income countries*. Geneva, World Health Organization, 2011 (http://www.who.int/nmh/publications/best_buys_summary.pdf, accessed 21 June 2013).

186. WHO Mental Health Gap Action Programme (mhGAP) [web site]. Geneva, World Health Organization, 2013 (http://www.who.int/mental_health/mhgap/en, accessed 21 June 2013).

187. *Disease and injury regional estimates: cause-specific mortality (2008 Global Burden of Disease)*. Geneva, World Health Organization, 2008 (http://www.who.int/healthinfo/global_burden_disease/estimates_regional/en/index.html, accessed 21 June 2013).

188. Sethi D et al. *Injuries and violence in Europe: why they matter and what can be done*. Copenhagen, WHO Regional Office for Europe, 2006 (http://www.euro.who.int/__data/assets/pdf_file/0005/98762/E88037.pdf, accessed 21 June 2013).

189. Mortality by 67 causes of death, age and sex [online database]. Copenhagen, WHO Regional Office for Europe, 2011 (http://www.euro.who.int/hfadb, accessed 21 June 2013).

190. Krug EG et al. *World report on violence and health*. Geneva, World Health Organization, 2002 (http://www.who.int/violence_injury_prevention/violence/world_report/en/index.html, accessed 21 June 2013).

191. Racioppi F et al. *Preventing road traffic injury: a public health perspective for Europe*. Copenhagen, WHO Regional Office for Europe, 2004 (http://www.euro.who.int/__data/assets/pdf_file/0003/87564/E82659.pdf, accessed 21 June 2013).

192. *Preventing injuries and violence. A guide for ministries of health*. Geneva, World Health Organization, 2007 (http://www.who.int/violence_injury_prevention/en, accessed 21 June 2013).

193. Sethi D et al. Reducing inequalities from injuries in Europe. *Lancet*, 2006, 368:2243–2250.

194. Sethi D et al. *Preventing injuries in Europe: from international collaboration to local implementation*. Copenhagen, WHO Regional Office for Europe, 2010 (http://www.euro.who.int/__data/assets/pdf_file/0011/96455/E93567.pdf, accessed 21 June 2013).

195. *WHO Regional Committee for Europe resolution EUR/RC55/R9 on the prevention of injuries.* Copenhagen, WHO Regional Office for Europe, 1995 (http://www.euro.who.int/__data/assets/pdf_file/0017/88100/RC55_eres09.pdf, accessed 21 June 2013).

196. *TEACH-VIP users' manual.* Geneva, World Health Organization, 2005 (http://www.who.int/violence_injury_prevention/capacitybuilding/teach_vip/en/index.html, accessed 21 June 2013).

197. Global Alert and Response (GAR): Global Outbreak Alert & Response Network [web site]. Geneva, World Health Organization, 2013 (http://www.who.int/csr/outbreaknetwork/en, accessed 21 June 2013).

198. Odolini S et al. Travel-related imported infections in Europe. *Clinical Microbiology and Infection,* 2012, 18:468–474.

199. *UNAIDS Report on the global AIDS epidemic.* Geneva, UNAIDS, 2010 (http://www.unaids.org/globalreport/documents/20101123_GlobalReport_full_en.pdf, accessed 21 June 2013).

200. European Centre for Disease Prevention and Control and WHO Regional Office for Europe. *HIV/AIDS surveillance in Europe 2009.* Stockholm, European Centre for Disease Prevention and Control, 2010 (http://www.ecdc.europa.eu/en/publications/publications/101129_sur_hiv_2009.pdf, accessed 21 June 2013).

201. European Centre for Disease Prevention and Control and WHO Regional Office for Europe. *Tuberculosis surveillance in Europe 2009.* Stockholm, European Centre for Disease Prevention and Control, 2011 (http://ecdc.europa.eu/en/publications/Publications/1103_TB_SUR_2009.pdf, accessed 21 June 2013).

202. Kardar SS. *Antibiotic resistance: new approaches to a historical problem.* Reston, VA, Action Bioscience, 2005.

203. Heymann DL, Rodier G. Global surveillance, national surveillance, and SARS. *Emerging Infectious Diseases*, 2004, 10:173–175.

204. *Communicable diseases and public policy.* Washington, DC, World Bank, 2007 (siteresources.worldbank.org/EXTABOUTUS/Resources/communicabledisease.ppt, accessed 21 June 2013).

205. *Immunization summary: a statistical reference containing data through 2009.* New York, UNICEF Statistics and Monitoring Section Division of Policy and Practice and Geneva, World Health Organization, 2011 (http://www.childinfo.org/files/32775_UNICEF.pdf, accessed 21 June 2013).

206. *Important changes to the childhood immunisation programme.* Brussels, European Cervical Cancer Association, 2009 (http://www.ecca.info/fileadmin/user_upload/HPV_Vaccination/ECCA_HPV_Vaccination_April_2009.pdf, accessed 21 June 2013).

207. Trotter CL, Ramsay ME, Slack MP. Rising incidence of *Haemophilus influenzae* type b disease in England and Wales indicates a need for a second catch-up vaccination campaign. *Communicable Disease and Public Health*, 2003, 6:55–58.

208. *Pneumococcal vaccine added to the childhood immunisation programme; more protection against meningitis and septicaemia.* London, Department of Health, 2006 (http://webarchive.nationalarchives.gov.uk/+/www.dh.gov.uk/en/Publicationsandstatistics/Pressreleases/DH_4128036, accessed 21 June 2013).

209. Meningococcal vaccines: polysaccharide and polysaccharide conjugate vaccines. *WHO Weekly Epidemiological Record*, 2002, 77:331–338.

210. European Immunization Week [web site]. Copenhagen, WHO Regional Office for Europe, 2013 (http://eiw.euro.who.int, accessed 21 June 2013).

211. Mankertz A et al. Molecular genotyping and epidemiology of measles virus transmission in the World Health Organization European Region, 2007–2009. *Journal of Infectious Diseases*, 2010, 204(Suppl 1):S335–S342.

212. Centralized Information System for Infectious Diseases [web site]. Copenhagen, WHO Regional Office for Europe, 2013 (http://data.euro.who.int/cisid, accessed 21 June 2013).

213. Laboratory Data Management System for Polio Laboratory Network [web site]. Copenhagen, WHO Regional Office for Europe, 2013 (http://ldms.euro.who.int, accessed 21 June 2013).

214. Shooter RA. *Report of the investigation into the cause of the 1978 Birmingham smallpox occurrence.* London, H.M. Stationery Office, 1980.

215. Lim PL et al. Laboratory-acquired severe acute respiratory syndrome. *New England Journal of Medicine*, 2004, 350:1740–1745.

216. Kumarasamy KK et al. Emergence of a new antibiotic resistance mechanism in India, Pakistan, and the United Kingdom: a molecular, biological, and epidemiological study. *Lancet Infectious Diseases*, 2010, 10:597–602.

217. *European strategic action plan on antibiotic resistance.* Copenhagen, WHO Regional Office for Europe, 2011 (http://www.euro.who.int/__data/assets/pdf_file/0008/147734/wd14E_AntibioticResistance_111380.pdf, accessed 21 June 2013).

218. Abubakar I et al. Tackling the spread of drug-resistant tuberculosis in Europe. *Lancet*, 2012, 379:e21–e23.

219. *Roadmap to prevent and combat drug-resistant tuberculosis. The Consolidated Action Plan to Prevent and Combat Multidrug- and Extensively Drug-Resistant Tuberculosis in the WHO European Region 2011–2015.* Copenhagen, WHO Regional Office for Europe, 2011 (http://www.euro.who.int/__data/assets/pdf_file/0014/152015/e95786.pdf, accessed 21 June 2013).

220. Abubakar I et al. *Rapid implementation of the Xpert MTB/RIF diagnostic test.* Geneva, World Health Organization, 2011 (http://whqlibdoc.who.int/publications/2011/9789241501569_eng.pdf, accessed 21 June 2013).

221. WHO, UNAIDS and UNICEF. *Towards universal access: scaling up priority HIV/AIDS interventions in the health sector. Progress report 2010.* Geneva, World Health Organization, 2010 (http://www.who.int/hiv/pub/2010progressreport/report/en/index.html, accessed 21 June 2013).

222. *European Action Plan for HIV/AIDS 2012–2015.* Copenhagen, WHO Regional Office for Europe, 2011 (http://www.euro.who.int/__data/assets/pdf_file/0011/153875/e95953.pdf, accessed 21 June 2013).

223. *What is quality improvement in HIV prevention?* Geneva, IQhiv, 2012 (http://iqhiv.org/get-started/what-is-it, accessed 21 June 2013).

224. Mirzoaliev I et al. [Efficiency of a package of therapeutic and preventive measures in the Republic of Tajikistan in the malaria postepidemic period (2000–2007)]. *Meditsinskaia Parazitologiia i parazitarnye bolezni (Moskva)*, 2009, 4:47–49.

225. Barbić L et al. Spreading of West Nile virus infection in Croatia. *Veterinary Microbiology*, 2012, 159:504–508.

226. Christodoulou V et al. Re-emergence of visceral and cutaneous leishmaniasis in the Greek island of Crete. *Vector-borne Zoonotic Diseases*, 2012, 12:214–222.

227. Ryan J et al. Establishing the health and economic impact of influenza vaccination within the European Union 25 countries. *Vaccine*, 2006, 24:6812–6822.

228. *How to become a WHO-recognized national influenza centre: guidance on the process for influenza laboratories in the WHO European Region*. Copenhagen, WHO Regional Office for Europe, 2012 (http://www.euro.who.int/__data/assets/pdf_file/0007/126457/e94432.pdf, accessed 21 June 2013).

229. *Recommendations for good practice in pandemic preparedness: identified through evaluation of the response to pandemic (H1N1) 2009*. Copenhagen, WHO Regional Office for Europe, 2012 (http://www.euro.who.int/__data/assets/pdf_file/0017/128060/e94534.pdf, accessed 21 June 2013).

230. Ritsatakis A, Makara P. *Gaining health. Analysis of policy development in European countries for tackling noncommunicable diseases*. Copenhagen, World Health Organization, 2009 (http://www.euro.who.int/__data/assets/pdf_file/0018/105318/e92828.pdf, accessed 21 June 2013).

231. Busse R et al. *Tackling chronic disease in Europe: strategies, interventions and challenges.* Copenhagen, World Health Organization on behalf of the European Observatory on Health Systems and Policies, 2010 (Observatory Studies Series, No. 20; http://www.euro.who.int/__data/assets/pdf_file/0008/96632/E93736.pdf, accessed 21 June 2013).

232. *WHO Regional Committee for Europe resolution EUR/RC58/R4. Stewardship/governance of health systems in the WHO European Region*. Copenhagen, World Health Organization, 2008 (http://www.euro.who.int/__data/assets/pdf_file/0016/70243/RC58_eres04.pdf, accessed 21 June 2013).

233. *European action plan for strengthening public health capacities and services*. Copenhagen, WHO Regional Office for Europe, 2012 (http://www.euro.who.int/__data/assets/pdf_file/0005/171770/RC62wd12rev1-Eng.pdf, accessed 21 June 2013).

234. Acheson D. *Public health in England: the report of the Committee of Inquiry into the Future Development of the Public Health Function*. London, H.M. Stationery Office, 1988.

235. *The world health report 2008 – Primary health care – now more than ever.* Geneva, World Health Organization, 2008 (http://www.who.int/whr/2008/en/index.html, accessed 21 June 2013).

236. *The WHO Global Code of Practice on the International Recruitment of Health Personnel.* Geneva, World Health Organization, 2010 (http://www.who.int/entity/hrh/migration/code/code_en.pdf, accessed 21 June 2013).

237. *The world health report 2010 – Health systems financing: the path to universal coverage.* Geneva, World Health Organization, 2010 (http://www.who.int/whr/2010/en/index.html, accessed 21 June 2013).

238. Kutzin J, Cashin C, Jakab S, eds. *Implementing health financing reform: lessons from countries in transition*. Copenhagen, World Health Organization on behalf of the European Observatory on Health Systems and Policies, 2010 (http://www.euro.who.int/__data/assets/pdf_file/0014/120164/E94240.pdf, accessed 21 June 2013).

239. Thomson S et al. *Addressing financial sustainability in health systems.* Copenhagen, World Health Organization on behalf of the European Observatory on Health Systems and Policies, 2010 (http://www.euro.who.int/__data/assets/pdf_file/0005/64949/E93058.pdf, accessed 21 June 2013).

240. Rodier G et al. Global public health security. *Emerging Infectious Diseases*, 2007, 13:1447–1452.

241. *International Health Regulations. IHR Core Capacity Monitoring Framework: checklist and indicators for monitoring progress in the development of IHR core capacities in States Parties.* Geneva, World Health Organization, 2010 (http://www.who.int/ihr/IHR_Monitoring_Framework_Checklist_and_Indicators.pdf, accessed 21 June 2013).

242. *Human development report 2011 – Human Development Index trends 1980–2011.* New York, United Nations Development Programme, 2011 (http://hdr.undp.org/en/reports/global/hdr2011/download, accessed 21 June 2013).

243. *Preventing disease through healthy environments. Towards an estimate of the environmental burden of diseases.* Geneva, World Health Organization, 2006 (http://www.who.int/quantifying_ehimpacts/publications/preventingdisease.pdf, accessed 21 June 2013).

244. *Health and environment in Europe: progress assessment.* Copenhagen, WHO Regional Office for Europe, 2010 (http://www.euro.who.int/__data/assets/pdf_file/0010/96463/E93556.pdf, accessed 21 June 2013).

245. *WHO guidelines on indoor air quality: dampness and mould.* Copenhagen, WHO Regional Office for Europe, 2009 (http://www.euro.who.int/__data/assets/pdf_file/0017/43325/E92645.pdf, accessed 21 June 2013).

246. *Burden of disease from environmental noise.* Copenhagen, WHO Regional Office for Europe, 2010 (http://www.euro.who.int/__data/assets/pdf_file/0008/136466/e94888.pdf, accessed 21 June 2013).

247. PCT databank on soil-transmitted helminthiasis [online database]. Geneva, World Health Organization, 2013 (http://www.who.int/neglected_diseases/preventive_chemotherapy/sth/db/index.html?units=minimal&region=EUR&country=all&countries=all&year=2010, accessed 21 June 2013).

248. *Progress on sanitation and drinking-water, 2010 update.* Geneva, World Health Organization, 2010 (http://whqlibdoc.who.int/publications/2010/9789241563956_eng_full_text.pdf, accessed 21 June 2013).

249. *Environmental health inequalities in Europe. Assessment report.* Copenhagen, WHO Regional Office for Europe, 2012 (http://www.euro.who.int/__data/assets/pdf_file/0010/157969/e96194.pdf, accessed 21 June 2013).

250. Lang T, Rayner G. Overcoming policy cacophony on obesity: an ecological public health framework for policymakers. *Obesity Reviews*, 2007, 8(Suppl. 1):165–181.

251. Morris G et al. Getting strategic about the environment and health. *Public Health*, 2006, 120:889–903.

252. *European environment outlook.* Copenhagen, European Environment Agency, 2005 (EEA Report no. 4/2005; http://www.eea.europa.eu/publications/eea_report_2005_4, accessed 21 June 2013).

253. Menne B et al. *Protecting health in Europe from climate change.* Copenhagen, WHO Regional Office for Europe, 2009 (http://www.euro.who.int/__data/assets/pdf_file/0016/74401/E91865.pdf, accessed 21 June 2013).

254. Stern N. *The economics of climate change: the Stern review.* Cambridge, Cambridge University Press, 2007.

255. European process on environment and health [web site]. Copenhagen, WHO Regional Office for Europe, 2013 (http://www.euro.who.int/en/what-we-do/health-topics/environment-and-health/european-process-on-environment-and-health/governance, accessed 21 June 2013).

256. *Protecting children's health in a changing environment. Report of the Fifth Ministerial Conference on Environment and Health*. Copenhagen, WHO Regional Office for Europe, 2010 (http://www.euro.who.int/__data/assets/pdf_file/0004/123565/e94331.pdf, accessed 21 June 2013).

257. *Regional report on the status of implementation of the Protocol on Water and Health to the Convention on the Protection and Use of Transboundary Watercourses and International Lakes. Second session of the Meeting of the Parties (Bucharest, 23–25 November 2010)*. Economic Commission for Europe and WHO Regional Office for Europe, 2010 (http://www.unece.org/fileadmin/DAM/env/documents/2010/wat/MP_WH/wh/ece_mp_wh_2010_2_E.pdf, accessed 21 June 2013).

258. United Nations Economic Commission for Europe et al., eds. *From transition to transformation: sustainable and inclusive development in Europe and central Asia*. Geneva, United Nations Economic Commission for Europe, 2012 (http://www.unep.org/roe/Portals/139/Moscow/From-Transition-to-Transformation.pdf, accessed 21 June 2013).

259. *Earth Summit. Agenda 21. The United Nations Programme for Action from Rio*. New York, United Nations, 1992 (http://www.un.org/esa/dsd/agenda21, accessed 21 June 2013).

260. *Rio Declaration on Environment and Sustainable Development*. New York, United Nations, 1992 (http://www.unep.org/Documents.Multilingual/Default.asp?documentid=78&articleid=1163).

261. *Global risks 2011*. 6th ed. Geneva, World Economic Forum, 2011.

262. *Sustainable development: from Brundtland to Rio 2012*. New York, United Nations, 2010 (http://www.un.org/wcm/webdav/site/climatechange/shared/gsp/docs/GSP1-6_Background%20on%20Sustainable%20Devt.pdf, accessed 21 June 2013).

263. Hosking J, Mudu P, Dora C. *Health co-benefits of climate change mitigation – transport sector*. Geneva, World Health Organization, 2012 (http://www.who.int/hia/examples/trspt_comms/hge_transport_lowresdurban_30_11_2011.pdf, accessed 21 June 2013).

264. *Health in the green economy: health co-benefits of climate change mitigation – housing sector*. Geneva, World Health Organization, 2011 (http://www.who.int/hia/hgehousing.pdf, accessed 21 June 2013).

265. United Nations, Department of Economic and Social Affairs, Population Division. *World urbanization prospects, the 2009 revision: highlights*. New York, United Nations, 2010.

266. Vlahov D et al., eds. *Urban health: global perspectives*. Hoboken, NJ, Wiley and Sons, 2010.

267. *Unmasking and overcoming health inequities in urban settings*. Geneva, World Health Organization, and UN-HABITAT, 2010.

268. Barton H et al. Healthy urban planning in European cities. *Health Promotion International*, 2009, 24:91–99.

269. Tsouros A. City leadership for health and sustainable development. *Health Promotion International*, 2009, 24:4–10.

270. Tsouros A, Green G, Healthy Cities: lessons learnt. In: Vlahov D et al., eds. *Urban health: global perspectives*. Hoboken, NJ, Wiley and Sons, 2010.

271. *Phase V (2009–2013) of the WHO European Healthy Cities Network: goals and requirements*. Copenhagen, WHO Regional Office for Europe, 2009 (http://www.euro.who.int/__data/assets/pdf_file/0009/100989/E92260.pdf, accessed 21 June 2013).

272. Gilson L et al. *Challenging inequity through health systems. Final report of the Knowledge Network on Health Systems of the Commission on the Social Determinants of Health*. Geneva, World Health Organization, 2007 (http://www.who.int/social_determinants/resources/csdh_media/hskn_final_2007_en.pdf, accessed 21 June 2013).

273. Morgan A, Davies M, Ziglio E. *Health assets in the global context*. London, Springer, 2010.

274. United Nations Secretary-General's High-level Panel on Global Sustainability. *Resilient people, resilient planet: a future worth choosing*. New York, United Nations, 2012.

275. *Assets Alliance Scotland*. Edinburgh, LTCAS, Scottish Community Development Centre and the Scottish Government, 2011 (http://www.scdc.org.uk/media/resources/news-and-events/Assets%20Alliance%20Scotland%20Event%2013%20Dec%202010%20Report.pdf, accessed 21 June 2013).

276. Strand M et al. *Setting the political agenda to tackle health inequity in Norway*. Copenhagen, WHO Regional Office for Europe, 2009 (http://www.euro.who.int/__data/assets/pdf_file/0014/110228/E93431.pdf, accessed 21 June 2013).

277. Lim SS et al. Prevention of cardiovascular disease in high-risk individuals in low-income and middle-income countries: health effects and costs, *Lancet*, 2007, 370:2054–2062.

278. Brown C et al. *Governance for SDH – appraisal tool*. Copenhagen, WHO Regional Office for Europe, 2010.

279. Antonovsky A. *Health, stress and coping*. San Francisco, Jossey-Bass, 1979.

280. Antonovsky A. *Unraveling the mystery of health. How people manage stress and stay well*. San Francisco, Jossey-Bass, 1987.

281. Morgan A, Ziglio E. Revitalizing the evidence base for public health: an assets model. *Promotion and Education*, 2007, 2(Suppl.):17–22.

282. *Living Well across communities: prioritizing well-being to reduce inequalities*. Manchester, NHS North West, 2010 (http://www.nwph.net/hawa/writedir/a862Living%20Well.pdf.pdf, accessed 21 June 2013).

283. Brown C, Buzeti T. *Placing social determinants of health on the regional development agenda: investment for health and development in Slovenia*. Copenhagen, WHO Regional Office for Europe, in press.

284. *A whole-of-government approach to reducing health inequalities: the Scottish experience*. Copenhagen, WHO Regional Office for Europe, in press.

285. Swanson D et al. Seven guidelines for policy making in its uncertain world. In: Swanson D, Bhadwal S, eds. *Creating adaptive policies: a guide for policy making in an uncertain world*. London, Sage, 2009.

286. European Innovation Partnership on Active and Healthy Ageing [web site]. Brussels, European Commission, 2013 (http://ec.europa.eu/research/innovation-union/index_en.cfm?section=active-healthy-ageing, accessed 21 June 2013).

287. Paquet G. The new governance: subsidiarity and the strategic state. In: *Governance in the 21st century*. Paris, Organisation for Economic Co-operation and Development, 2001.

288. HealthyPeople.gov [web site]. Washington, DC, United States Department of Health and Human Services, 2013 (http://healthypeople.gov/2020/default.aspx, accessed 21 June 2013).

289. Brown C et al. *Governance for health equity and the social determinants of health – a companion resource to support national review*. Copenhagen, WHO Regional Office for Europe (forthcoming).

290. Brown C. *Progress and opportunities in implementing health in all policies – a rapid appraisal of learning from Europe and internationally*. Copenhagen, WHO Regional Office for Europe (forthcoming).

291. Harrison D et al. *Report of the Task Group on Governance and Delivery Mechanisms*. Copenhagen, WHO Regional Office for Europe (forthcoming).

292. Marks L. Accountability for social determinants of health and health equity. In: Brown C et al. *Governance for health equity and the social determinants of health – a companion resource to support national review*. Copenhagen, WHO Regional Office for Europe (forthcoming).

293. *South Australia's Strategic Plan: progress report*. Adelaide, South Australia's Strategic Plan Audit Committee, 2010.

294. McDaid D. Joint budgeting: can it facilitate intersectoral action? In: McQueen D et al., eds. *Intersectoral governance for health in all policies: structures, actions and experiences*. Copenhagen, World Health Organization on behalf of the European Observatory on Health Systems and Policies, 2012 (http://www.euro.who.int/__data/assets/pdf_file/0005/171707/intersectoral-governance-for-health-in-all-policies.pdf, accessed 21 June 2013).

295. *Communication from the Commission to the European Parliament, the Council, the European Economic and Social Committee and the Committee of the Regions: an EU framework for national Roma integration strategies up to 2020*. Brussels, European Commission, 2011 (COM(2011) 173 final).

296. Dahlgren G, Whitehead M. *European strategies for tackling social inequities in health: levelling up part 2*. Copenhagen, WHO Regional Office for Europe, 2007 (Studies on Social and Economic Determinants of Population Health, No. 3; http://www.euro.who.int/__data/assets/pdf_file/0018/103824/E89384.pdf, accessed 21 June 2013).

297. *Biennial report 2008–2009 and key developments for 2010–2011 of the WHO European Office for Investment for Health and Development*. Copenhagen, WHO Regional Office for Europe, 2011.

298. Brown C, Ziglio E, Rohregger B. *Appraisal of governance systems and capacity for addressing social determinants of health and health equity*. Copenhagen, WHO Regional Office for Europe (forthcoming).

299. *Report on the 3rd Ministerial Meeting of the Countries of the South-Eastern Europe Health Network – opportunities for scaling up and strengthening health in all policies in south-eastern Europe*. Copenhagen, WHO Regional Office for Europe (forthcoming).

300. Blas E, Sivisankara KA, eds. *Equity, social determinants and public health programmes*. Geneva, World Health Organization, 2011 (http://www.who.int/social_determinants/en, accessed 21 June 2013).

301. Blas E, Sommerfeld J, Sivasankara AK, eds. *Social determinants approaches to public health: from concept to practice*. Geneva, World Health Organization, 2011 (http://www.who.int/social_determinants/en, accessed 21 June 2013).

302. Bertollini R, Brassart C, Galanaki C. *Review of the commitments of WHO European Member States and the WHO Regional Office for Europe between 1990 and 2010. Analysis in the light of the Health 2020 strategy*. Copenhagen, WHO Regional Office for Europe, 2012 (http://www.euro.who.int/__data/assets/pdf_file/0020/171902/Review-of-the-commitments-of-WHO-European-Member-States-and-the-WHO-Regional-Office-for-Europe-between-1990-and-2010.pdf, accessed 21 June 2013).

Annex. Glossary of working definitions and explanatory notes on concepts and terms used in Health 2020

Determinants of health

This term refers to the range of personal, social, economic and environmental factors that determine the health status of individuals or population.

Commission on Social Determinants of Health. *Closing the gap in a generation: health equity through action on the social determinants of health. Final report of the Commission on Social Determinants of Health*. Geneva, World Health Organization, 2008 (http://www.who.int/social_determinants/resources/gkn_lee_al.pdf, accessed 21 June 2013).

Empowerment

Empowerment covers a very wide range of meanings, definitions and interpretations. In general, the term is about the ability to make decisions about personal and collective circumstances. In the context of Health 2020, empowerment is a process through which people gain greater control over decisions and actions affecting their health. To achieve this, individuals and communities need to develop skills, have access to information and resources, and opportunities to have a voice and influence the factors affecting their health and well-being.

Adapted and expanded from: *Health promotion glossary*. Geneva, World Health Organization, 1998 (http://www.who.int/healthpromotion/about/HPR%20Glossary%201998.pdf).

Essential public health operations

The fundamental operations that must be carried out in society in order to maximize the health and well-being of the population as well as health equity. In the European Region of WHO, these are: (i) surveillance of population health and well-being; (ii) monitoring of and response to health hazards and emergencies; (iii) health protection, including environmental, occupational, food safety and others; (iv) health promotion, including action to address social determinants and health inequity; (v) disease prevention, including early detection of illness; (vi) assuring governance for health and well-being; (vii) assuring a sufficient and competent public health workforce; (viii) assuring sustainable organizational structures and financing; (ix) advocacy, communication and social mobilization for health; and (x) advancing public health research to inform policy and practice.

European Action Plan for Strengthening Public Health Capacities and Services. Copenhagen, WHO Regional Office for Europe, 2012 (document EUR/RC62/12).

Gender equity in health

Gender equity refers to fairness and justice in the distribution of benefits, power, resources and responsibilities between women and men to allow them to attain their full health potential. The concept recognizes that women and men have different needs and opportunities that impact on their health status, their access to services and their contributions to the health workforce. It acknowledges that these differences should be identified and addressed in a manner that rectifies the imbalance between the sexes.

Adapted from: *Mainstreaming gender equity in health: the need to move forward (Madrid Statement)*. Copenhagen, WHO Regional Office for Europe, 2002 (http://www.euro.who.int/__data/assets/pdf_file/0008/76508/A75328.pdf).
Gender mainstreaming for health managers: a practical approach. Geneva, World Health Organization, 2011 (http://www.who.int/gender/mainstreaming/tools/en/index1.html).

Governance

Governance is about how governments and other social organizations interact, how they relate to citizens, and how decisions are taken in a complex and globalized world.

Graham J, Amos B, Plumptre T. *Principles for good governance in the 21st century.* Ottawa, Institute on Governance, 2003 (Policy Brief No.15, http://unpan1.un.org/intradoc/groups/public/documents/UNPAN/UNPAN011842.pdf).

Governance for health

The attempts of governments and other actors to steer communities, countries or groups of countries in the pursuit of health as integral to well-being through both whole-of-government and whole-of-society approaches.

Kickbusch I, Gleicher D. *Governance for health in the 21st century*. Copenhagen, WHO Regional Office for Europe, 2012 (http://www.euro.who.int/__data/assets/pdf_file/0019/171334/RC62BD01-Governance-for-Health-Web.pdf, accessed 21 June 2013).

Health

A state of complete physical, mental and social well-being and not merely the absence of disease or infirmity.

Constitution of the World Health Organization. Geneva, World Health Organization, 1946 (Official Records of the World Health Organization, no. 2, p. 100; http://apps.who.int/gb/bd/PDF/bd47/EN/constitution-en.pdf).

Health asset

At a broad level, a health asset can be defined as any factor (or resource) that enhances the ability of individuals, communities and populations to protect, promote and sustain their health and well-being. These assets can operate at the level of individual, group, community, and/or population as protective factors to buffer against life's stresses and as promoting factors to maximize opportunities for health.

Adapted from: Ziglio E et al. *Maximizing health potential: the asset model for health and development*. Copenhagen, WHO Regional Office for Europe (forthcoming).

Health equity (and equity in health)

Equity is the absence of avoidable, unfair, or remediable differences among groups of people, whether those groups are defined socially, economically, demographically or geographically. "Health equity" or "equity in health" implies that ideally everyone should have a fair opportunity to attain their full health potential and, more pragmatically, that no one should be disadvantaged from achieving this potential.

Health systems topics – Equity [web site]. Geneva, World Health Organization, 2012. (http://www.who.int/healthsystems/topics/equity/en) and Glossary: Health equity [web site]. Copenhagen, WHO Regional Office for Europe, 2012 (http://www.euro.who.int/observatory/Glossary/TopPage?phrase=Equity).

Health for All

A policy goal consisting in the attainment by all the people of the world of a level of health that will permit them to lead a socially and economically productive life.

Adapted from: *Glossary of terms used in Health for All series*. Geneva, World Health Organization, 1984.

Health governance

The governance of the health system and health system strengthening.

Kickbusch I, Gleicher D. *Governance for health in the 21st century*. Copenhagen, WHO Regional Office for Europe, 2012 (http://www.euro.who.int/__data/assets/pdf_file/0019/171334/RC62BD01-Governance-for-Health-Web.pdf, accessed 21 June 2013).

Health in all policies

There are numerous definitions of the term Health in All Policies, basically focusing on the need to incorporate an explicit concern for health in the policies of all sectors. In the context of Health 2020, a Health in All Policies approach is designed to make governance for health and well-being a priority for more than the health sector. It works in both directions, ensuring that all sectors understand and act on their responsibility for health, while recognizing how health affects other sectors. The health sector can therefore, support other arms of government by actively assisting their policy development and goal attainment.

To harness health and well-being, governments need institutionalized processes that value cross-sector problem-solving and address power imbalances. This includes providing the leadership, mandate, incentives, budgetary commitment and sustainable mechanisms that support government agencies to work collaboratively on integrated solutions.

> Adapted from: *Adelaide Statement on Health in All Policies*. Geneva, World Health Organization, 2010 (http://www.who.int/social_determinants/hiap_statement_who_sa_final.pdf).

Health inequality

The term means a difference in health status between individuals or groups, as measured by, for example, life expectancy, mortality or disease. Health inequalities are the differences, variations and disparities in the health achievements of individuals and groups of people. Some differences are due to biological or other unavoidable factors such as age; others, however, are avoidable.

> Kawachi I. A glossary for health inequalities. Journal of Epidemiology and Community Health, 2002, 56:647.

Health inequity

Health inequity refers to a difference or inequality in health that is deemed to be avoidable, unfair or stemming from some form of injustice. Inequities in health status can be between groups of people within countries and or between countries. Health inequities arise from differences within and between societies and the distribution of resources and power. Inequities are those differences in health that arise not from chance or from the decision of the individual but from avoidable differences in social, economic and environmental variables (such as living and working conditions, education, occupation, income and access to quality health care, disease prevention and health promotion services) that are largely beyond individual control and that can be addressed by public policy.

It should be noted that the terms *health inequalities* and *health inequities* are often used interchangeably, while in most languages other than English there is only one term to describe such differences. Thus the term *health inequalities* is also used to refer to those differences in health that are deemed to be avoidable and unfair and that are strongly influenced by the actions of governments, stakeholders and communities, and that can be addressed by public policy. Therefore the terms *health inequality* and *health inequity* are commonly used to refer to those health differences that are unfair and avoidable.

> Kawachi I. A glossary for health inequalities. *Journal of Epidemiology and Community Health*, 2002, 56:647.
>
> Commission on Social Determinants of Health. *Closing the gap in a generation: health equity through action on the social determinants of health*. Final report of the Commission on Social Determinants of Health. Geneva, World Health Organization, 2008 (http://whqlibdoc.who.int/publications/2008/9789241563703_eng.pdf).
>
> *Memo: questions and answers on solidarity in health: reducing health inequalities in the EU*. Brussels, Commission of the European Communities, 2009 (http://ec.europa.eu/health/ph_determinants/socio_economics/documents/com2009_qa_en.pdf).

Health literacy

The cognitive and social skills that determine the motivation and ability of individuals to gain access to, understand and use information in ways that promote and maintain good health.

Health promotion glossary. Geneva, World Health Organization, 1998 (http://www.who.int/healthpromotion/about/HPR%20Glossary%201998.pdf).

Health system

The ensemble of all public and private organizations, institutions and resources mandated to improve, maintain or restore health. Health systems encompass both personal and population services, as well as activities to influence the policies and actions of other sectors to address the social, environmental and economic determinants of health.

The Tallinn Charter: Health Systems for Health and Wealth. Copenhagen, WHO Regional Office for Europe, 2008 (http://www.euro.who.int/__data/assets/pdf_file/0008/88613/E91438.pdf).

Intersectoral action

This term refers to efforts by the health sector to work collaboratively with other sectors of society to achieve improved health outcomes.

Kickbusch I, Buckett K, eds *Implementing health in all policies.* Adelaide 2010. Adelaide, Department of Health, Government of South Australia, 2010 (http://www.who.int/sdhconference/resources/implementinghiapadel-sahealth-100622.pdf).

Life-course approach

This approach suggests that the health outcomes of individuals and the community depend on the interaction of multiple protective and risk factors throughout people's lives. The life-course approach provides a more comprehensive vision of health and its determinants and a focus on interventions in each stage of their lives.

Health System Strengthening Glossary [web site]. Geneva, World Health Organization, 2013 (http://www.who.int/healthsystems/hss_glossary/en/index6.html).

Adapted from: Lu M, Halfon N. Racial and ethnic disparities in birth outcomes: a life-course perspective. *Maternal and Child Health Journal* 2003, 7(1):13–30.

Primary health care

Essential health care made accessible at a cost that a country and community can afford, with methods that are practical, scientifically sound and socially acceptable.

Declaration of Alma-Ata. International Conference on Primary Health Care, Alma-Ata, USSR, 6–12 September 1978. Geneva, World Health Organization, 1978 (http://www.who.int/publications/almaata_declaration_en.pdf).

Public health

The science and art of preventing disease, prolonging life and promoting health through the organized efforts of society.

Acheson D. *Public health in England. The report of the committee of inquiry into the future development of the public health function.* London, HMSO, 1988.

Public health capacity

The resources (natural, financial, human or other) required to undertake the delivery of essential public health operations.

Developing a framework for action for strengthening public health capacities and services in Europe. Copenhagen, WHO Regional Office for Europe, 2011 (document EUR/RC61/Inf.Doc./1; http://www.euro.who.int/__data/assets/pdf_file/0009/148266/RC61_einfdoc01.pdf).

Public health services

The services involved in delivery of the essential public health operations. These services can be provided within the health system or in other sectors (beyond the strict boundaries of the health system) with health generating activities.

Developing a framework for action for strengthening public health capacities and services in Europe. Copenhagen, WHO Regional Office for Europe, 2011 (document EUR/RC61/Inf. Doc./1; http://www.euro.who.int/__data/assets/pdf_file/0009/148266/RC61_einfdoc01.pdf).

Resilience

The dynamic process of adapting well and responding individually or collectively in the face of challenging circumstances, economic crisis, psychological stress, trauma, tragedy, threats, and other significant sources of stress. It can be described as an ability to withstand, to cope or to recover from the effects of such circumstances and the process of identifying assets and enabling factors. Health 2020 places particular emphasis on the importance of creating resilient communities and the idea of helping people to help themselves. The term "resilient communities" is also frequently used in the context of disaster risk reduction (such as flooding) and the importance of creating appropriate infrastructures, systems and decision-making processes.

Derived from: Resilience [web site]. London, The Young Foundation, 2013 (http://www.youngfoundation.org/our-ventures?current_venture=2036). *Community resilience and co-production. Getting to grips with the language. A briefing paper*. Edinburgh, Scottish Community Development Centre, 2011 (http://www.scdc.org.uk/media/resources/assets-alliance/Community%20Resilience%20and%20Coproduction%20SCDC%20briefing%20paper.pdf) and *Empowering lives,building resilience. Development stories from Europe and central Asia*. Volume 1. New York, United Nations Development Programme, 2011 (http://www.undp.org/content/dam/undp/library/Cross-Practice%20generic%20theme/RBEC_Empowering%20Lives%20Building%20Resilience.pdf).

Social capital

Social capital represents the degree of social cohesion that exists in communities. It refers to the processes between people that establish networks, norms and social trust, and which facilitate coordination and cooperation for mutual benefits..

Health promotion glossary. Geneva, World Health Organization, 1998 (http://www.who.int/hpr/NPH/docs/hp_glossary_en.pdf).

Social determinants of health

The social determinants of health are the conditions in which people are born, grow, live, work and age, including the health system. These circumstances are shaped by the distribution of money, power and resources at global, national and local levels, which are themselves influenced by policy choices. The social determinants of health are mostly responsible for health inequities – the unfair and avoidable differences in health status seen within and between countries.

Commission on Social Determinants of Health. *Closing the gap in a generation: health equity through action on the social determinants of health. Final report of the Commission on Social Determinants of Health*. Geneva, World Health Organization, 2008 (http://whqlibdoc.who.int/publications/2008/9789241563703_eng.pdf).

Social gradient in health

The stepwise fashion in which health outcomes improve as socioeconomic position improves. This gradient can be measured by a person's income, occupation, or the highest level of education he or she has. Similarly, social gradient in health can be defined as the stepwise or linear decrease in health that comes with decreasing social position.

Kawachi I. *A glossary for health inequalities. Journal of Epidemiology and Community Health*, 2002, 56:647.

Marmot M. *The status syndrome: how social standing affects our health and longevity*. London, Bloomsbury Publishing PLC, 2004.

Social inequalities

Social inequalities refer to differences in the distribution of social and economic factors or the social determinants of health within a country and or between countries. Social inequalities are usually measured by income, education and occupation. These social inequalities contribute to differences in health status (health inequalities) and are often the primary source or cause of health inequalities. Action on health inequalities therefore also requires action on social determinants such as education, living and working conditions, employment and income. For example, joint action by the health and education sectors to ensure that young women remain at school and complete secondary education will improve their health and life opportunities and reduce the health and social inequalities related to lower levels of education or incomplete schooling.

Social network

Social relations and links between individuals which may provide access to or mobilization of social support for health.

Health promotion glossary. Geneva, World Health Organization, 1998 (http://www.who.int/hpr/NPH/docs/hp_glossary_en.pdf).

Sustainability

The capacity to endure. In environmental and development circles, the terms "sustainability" and "sustainable development" are often used interchangeably. The most widely cited definition of "sustainable development" is that of the World Commission on Environment and Development, which defined it as development that "meets the needs of the present without compromising the ability of future generations to meet their own needs". In health economics, the term sustainability is also employed to designate the potential for sustaining beneficial health outcomes for an agreed period at an acceptable level of resource commitment within acceptable organizational and community contingencies. Increasingly, efforts are being made to highlight the synergies between the public health and sustainability policy agendas.

Report of the World Commission on Environment and Development. General Assembly Resolution A/RES/42/187, 11 December 1987. New York, United Nations, 1987 (http://www.un.org/documents/ga/res/42/ares42-187.htm/).

Health System Strengthening Glossary [web site]. Geneva, World Health Organization, 2013 (http://www.who.int/healthsystems/hss_glossary/en/index6.html).

Well-being

Well-being is an integral part of the WHO definition of health: "Health is a state of complete physical, mental and social well-being and not merely the absence of disease or infirmity". It exists in two dimensions, subjective and objective. It comprises an individual's experience of his or her life, and a comparison of life circumstances with social norms and values. Subjective well-being can include a person's overall sense of well-being, psychological functioning, as well as affective states. Examples of objective well-being and life circumstances include health, education, jobs, social relationships, environment (built and natural), security, civic engagement and governance, housing and leisure.

Constitution of the World Health Organization. Geneva, World Health Organization, 1946 (Official Records of the World Health Organization, no. 2, p. 100; http://apps.who.int/gb/bd/PDF/bd47/EN/constitution-en.pdf).

Measurement of and target-setting for well-being: an initiative by the WHO Regional Office for Europe. First meeting of the expert group, Copenhagen, Denmark, 8–9 February 2012. Copenhagen, WHO Regional Office for Europe, 2012.

Whole-of-government approach

"Whole-of–government" refers to the diffusion of governance vertically across levels of government and arenas of governance and horizontally throughout sectors. Whole-of-government activities are multilevel, encompassing government activities and actors from local to global levels, and increasingly also involving groups outside government. Health in all policies is one whole-of-government approach to making governance for health and well-being a priority for more than the health sector, working in both directions: taking account of the impact of other sectors on health and the impact of health on other sectors.

Kickbusch I, Gleicher D. *Governance for health in the 21st century*. Copenhagen, WHO Regional Office for Europe, 2012 (http://www.euro.who.int/__data/assets/pdf_file/0019/171334/RC62BD01-Governance-for-Health-Web.pdf, accessed 21 June 2013).

Whole-of-society approach

"Whole-of-society" refers to an approach that aims to extend the whole-of-government approach by placing additional emphasis on the roles of the private sector and civil society, as well as of political decision-makers such as parliamentarians. By engaging the private sector, civil society, communities and individuals, the whole-of-society approach can strengthen the resilience of communities to withstand threats to their health, security and well-being. A whole-of-society approach goes beyond institutions: it influences and mobilizes local and global culture and media, rural and urban communities and all relevant policy sectors, such as the education system, the transport sector, the environment and even urban design.

Kickbusch I, Gleicher D. *Governance for health in the 21st century*. Copenhagen, WHO Regional Office for Europe, 2012 (http://www.euro.who.int/__data/assets/pdf_file/0019/171334/RC62BD01-Governance-for-Health-Web.pdf, accessed 21 June 2013).